Handbook of Pharmacology for
Nursing Students

AF067497

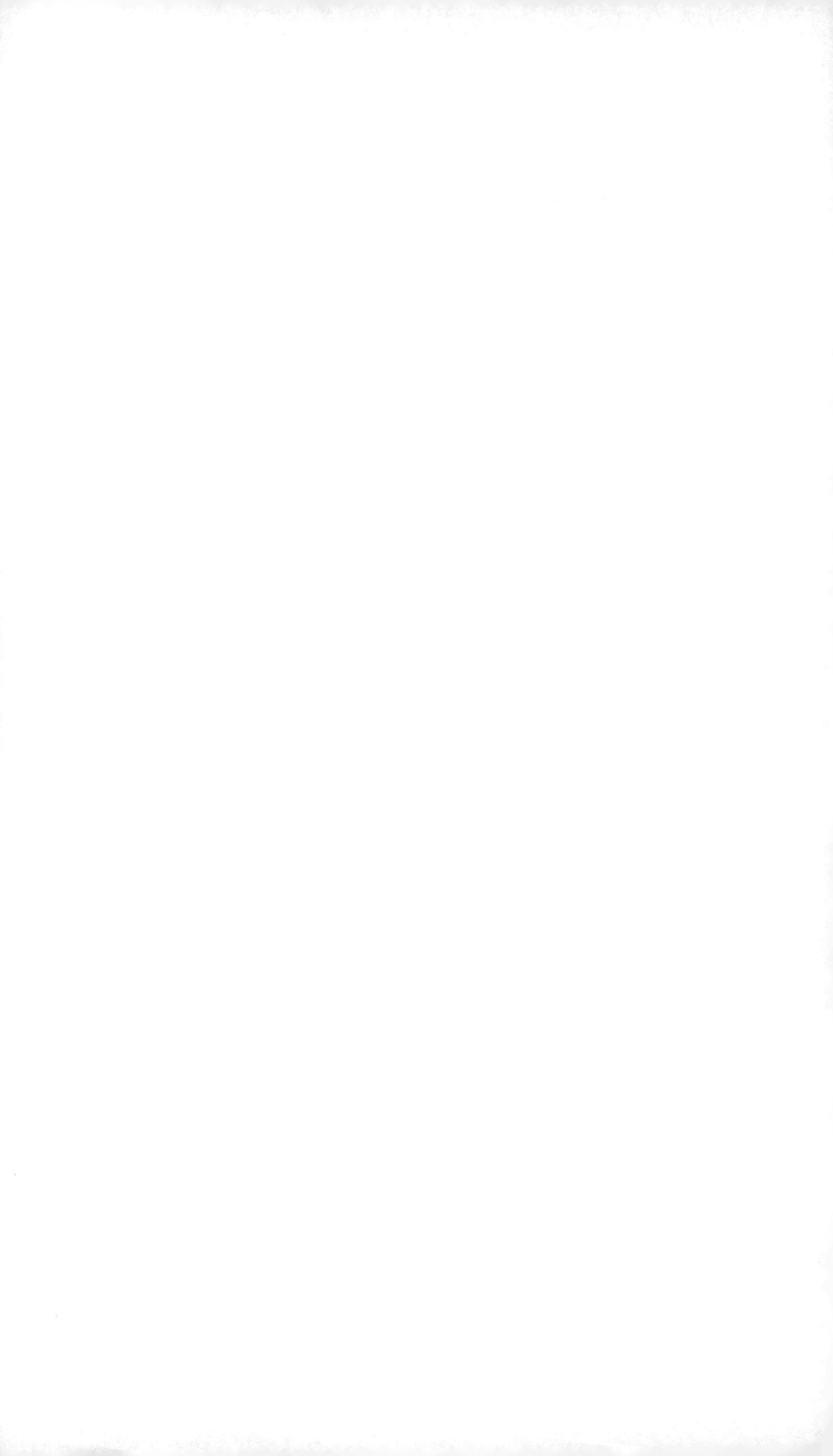

Handbook of Pharmacology for Nursing Students

Second Edition

Keshab Raj Paudel MD
Associate Professor and Course Director of Pharmacology
Trinity Medical Sciences University, St. Vincent and The Grenadines

Former Associate Professor of Pharmacology
Chitwan Medical College and Teaching Hospital
(Tribhuvan University), Chitwan, Nepal

Former Assistant Professor of Pharmacology
Kathmandu Medical College and Teaching Hospital
(Kathmandu University), Kathmandu, Nepal

Former Resident in Clinical Pharmacology and Therapeutics
BP Koirala Institute of Health Sciences, Dharan, Nepal
(Autonomous Health University)

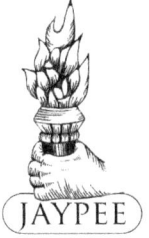

JAYPEE BROTHERS MEDICAL PUBLISHERS
The Health Sciences Publisher
New Delhi | London

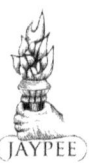 **Jaypee Brothers Medical Publishers (P) Ltd**

Headquarters

Jaypee Brothers Medical Publishers (P) Ltd
EMCA House, 23/23-B
Ansari Road, Daryaganj
New Delhi 110 002, India
Landline: +91-11-23272143, +91-11-23272703
+91-11-23282021, +91-11-23245672
Email: jaypee@jaypeebrothers.com

Corporate Office

Jaypee Brothers Medical Publishers (P) Ltd
4838/24, Ansari Road, Daryaganj
New Delhi 110 002, India
Phone: +91-11-43574357
Fax: +91-11-43574314
Email: jaypee@jaypeebrothers.com

Overseas Office

J.P. Medical Ltd
83 Victoria Street, London
SW1H 0HW (UK)
Phone: +44 20 3170 8910
Fax: +44 (0)20 3008 6180
Email: info@jpmedpub.com

Website: www.jaypeebrothers.com
Website: www.jaypeedigital.com

© 2022, Jaypee Brothers Medical Publishers

The views and opinions expressed in this book are solely those of the original contributor(s)/author(s) and do not necessarily represent those of editor(s) of the book.

All rights reserved. No part of this publication may be reproduced, stored or transmitted in any form or by any means, electronic, mechanical, photocopying, recording or otherwise, without the prior permission in writing of the publishers.

All brand names and product names used in this book are trade names, service marks, trademarks or registered trademarks of their respective owners. The publisher is not associated with any product or vendor mentioned in this book.

Medical knowledge and practice change constantly. This book is designed to provide accurate, authoritative information about the subject matter in question. However, readers are advised to check the most current information available on procedures included and check information from the manufacturer of each product to be administered, to verify the recommended dose, formula, method and duration of administration, adverse effects and contraindications. It is the responsibility of the practitioner to take all appropriate safety precautions. Neither the publisher nor the author(s)/editor(s) assume any liability for any injury and/or damage to persons or property arising from or related to use of material in this book.

This book is sold on the understanding that the publisher is not engaged in providing professional medical services. If such advice or services are required, the services of a competent medical professional should be sought.

Every effort has been made where necessary to contact holders of copyright to obtain permission to reproduce copyright material. If any have been inadvertently overlooked, the publisher will be pleased to make the necessary arrangements at the first opportunity.

Inquiries for bulk sales may be solicited at: jaypee@jaypeebrothers.com

Handbook of Pharmacology for Nursing Students

First Edition: 2014
Second Edition: **2022**
ISBN: 978-93-90595-26-6

Preface to the Second Edition

Handbook of Pharmacology for Nursing Students has been designed for Bachelor of Science (BSc) in Nursing incorporating different curricula under different universities as far as possible so that students can get every topic in this book and they do not have to wander for other books in the library or book stores. Another care that has been taken into consideration while preparing this book is to make the contents as much condensed and informative as possible. Therefore, both students and teachers can have the review of the relevant contents in short time to memorize the important information without pondering into unnecessary details.

Different chapters have been presented in brief with adequate information required for the course. Hopefully, the approach of writing this book was to help students to avoid overloaded information, yet empowering them with pertinent knowledge in Pharmacology without missing much needed information. The concept of this book came because of many subjects which have to be learnt in short time period for the students. So, reading more textual or contextual book necessitates more dedicated time, concentration and analysis than reading concise and informative books for undergraduates. This is the first endeavor to have the pharmacology book in this kind of format for the students. After the successful outcome of the first edition in 2014, second edition has been prepared incorporating readers feedback. Every chapter has been updated to keep abreast with recent advancements, discoveries and guidelines in the treatment approaches. New contents have been added in ANS, antidiabetic drugs, monoclonal antibodies, drug-food and drug-drug interactions, etc., due to increasing expansion and significance of these topics in clinical arena. Moreover, all the valued readers, students and teachers are most welcome for their genuine comments and constructive criticisms for the betterment of this book in the upcoming editions.

You are kindly requested to drop any kind of comments or suggestions at keshabpaudel@gmail.com.

Keshab Raj Paudel

Preface to the First Edition

Handbook of Pharmacology for Nursing Students has been designed for Bachelor of Science in Nursing incorporating different curricula under different universities as far as possible so that students can get every topic in this book itself and they don't have to wander for other books in the library or book stores. Another care that has been considered while preparing this book, is to make the contents as much as condensed and informative. So, both students and teachers can have the review of the contents in short time to memorize the important information.

Different chapters have been presented in brief with adequate information required for the course. Hopefully, this will enable the students to avoid overloaded information, yet without missing much needed information in pharmacology subject. The concept of this book came because of many subjects which have to be learnt in short time for the students. Thus, reading more textual or contextual book necessitates more dedicated time, concentration and analysis than reading concise and informative books for undergraduates. This is the first endeavor to have the pharmacology book in this kind of format for the students. So, all the valued readers, students and teachers are most welcome for their genuine comments and constructive criticisms for the betterment of this book in the upcoming editions.

You are kindly requested to drop any kind of comments or suggestions for *Handbook of Pharmacology for Nursing Students* at keshabpaudel@gmail.com.

Keshab Raj Paudel

Acknowledgments

I wish to express my high regard for those authors, editors, scientists and publishers whose book/work/articles I consulted during the time of manuscript preparation, without which preparation of this book would not have been possible. So, I want to express my heartfelt sincere respect to all who have contributed to the field of Pharmacology and helped to modernize and update science of drugs in this modern era.

I am very grateful to the whole team of M/s Jaypee Brothers Medical Publishers (P) Ltd, New Delhi, India, Shri Jitendar P Vij (Group Chairman), Mr Ankit Vij (Managing Director), Mr MS Mani (Group President), Dr Madhu Choudhary (Publishing Head-Education), Ms Pooja Bhandari (Production Head), Ms Sunita Katla (Executive Assistant to Group Chairman and Publishing Manager), Ms Samina Khan (Executive Assistant to Publishing Head-Education), Ms Dolly Dominic (Development Editor), Mr Rajesh Sharma (Production Coordinator), Ms Seema Dogra (Cover Visualizer) for all their support to work in this project and make it a success. Without their cooperation, I could not have completed this project.

I would like to extend my sincere gratitude to Mr Amit Khadka, Mr Suman Samanta, Mr S Hazra, and to the staff of Jaypee Brothers Medical Publishers (P) Limited, Kolkata Branch for their continuous support to the publication of this book. Besides, I want to express my deep appreciation and gratitude to Ms Shilpi Dutta for her copy-editing and timely communication during the publication process.

Finally, I am grateful to my wife and daughter, and the family for their continuous support and encouragement for the preparation of the manuscript of the book.

Contents

1. Basic Concepts ... 1
- Introduction to Pharmacology and its Terminology *1*
- Different Sources of Drugs *2*
- Different Dosage Forms of the Drugs *4*
- Implementation of Pharmacology in Nursing Practice *5*
- Routes of Drug Administration *7*
- Prescription Writing and Common Abbreviations *9*
- Pharmacokinetics *12*
- Pharmacodynamics *17*
- Factors Modifying Drug's Action *22*
- Adverse Drug Reaction *23*
- Therapeutic Drug Monitoring *25*
- Essential Drugs *27*
- Rational Use of Drugs *28*
- Drug Interactions *29*
- Cancer Chemotherapy *30*
- Antimicrobial Agents (AMAS) and Basic Principles of Antimicrobial Chemotherapy *33*
- Sulfonamides and Cotrimoxazole (Folate Antagonists) and Quinolones and Fluoroquinoloes (DNA Synthesis Inhibitors) *36*
- Cell Wall Synthesis Inhibitors—Penicillin, Cephalosporin, and Vancomycin *41*
- Protein Synthesis Inhibitors—Tetracycline, Chloramphenicol, Aminoglycosides, and Macrolides *45*
- Antiseptics and Disinfectants *49*
- Common Poisons and Antidotes *50*
- Chelating Agents *51*
- Vitamins, Vaccines, and Antisera *53*

2. Blood ... 60
- Hematinics Used in Anemia *60*
- Antimalarial Drugs *61*

- Drugs for Visceral Leishmaniasis (Kala-azar) and Filariasis *63*
- Drugs Affecting Coagulation and Bleeding *64*

3. Respiratory System   69

- Drugs Used in Bronchial Asthma, Chronic Obstructive Pulmonary Disease and Cough *69*
- Antitubercular Drugs *73*
- Histamine and Antihistamines *79*
- Nasal Decongestants *83*

4. Musculoskeletal System   84

- Nonsteroidal Anti-inflammatory Drugs (NSAIDs) *84*
- Drugs Used in the Treatment of Rheumatoid Arthritis and Gout *87*
- Skeletal Muscle Relaxants *90*

5. Cardiovascular System   94

- Hypertension *94*
- Antianginal Drugs *98*
- Treatment of Congestive Cardiac Failure (CCF) *101*
- Drugs Used in Rheumatic Fever and Myocardial Infarction *103*
- Antiarrhythmic Drugs *105*
- Treatment of Shock *108*

6. Urinary System   112

- Urinary Antiseptics and Drugs for Urinary Tract Infection *112*
- Important Nephrotoxic Drugs *113*

7. Endocrine System   114

- Pituitary Hormones *114*
- Insulin *122*
- Oral Antidiabetic Agents *124*
- Pharmacology of Corticosteroids *126*
- Thyroid Hormones and Antithyroid Drugs *128*

Contents **xiii**

- Drugs Acting on Uterine Musculature
  (Oxytocics and Tocolytics)   *130*
- Pharmacology of Male and Female Sex Hormones   *131*
- Methods of Contraception   *134*
- Treatment of Sexually Transmitted Diseases   *138*
- Anabolic Steroids   *141*
- Calcification and Bone Turnover: Parathormone
  (Parathyroid Hormone), Vitamin D, and Calcitonin   *141*

8. Gastrointestinal and Hepatobiliary System   145

- Drugs Used in Peptic Ulcer   *145*
- Emetics and Antiemetics   *146*
- Drugs Used in Constipation and Diarrhea   *147*
- Antiamoebic and Antiprotozoal Drugs   *150*
- Anthelmintics   *151*
- Common Antispasmodics   *156*
- Important Hepatotoxic Drugs   *156*

9. Autonomic Nervous System   157

- Cholinergic and Anticholinergic Drugs   *157*
- Adrenergic Drugs and Antiadrenergic Drugs   *162*
- Mydriatics and Miotics   *165*
- Local Anesthetic Agents   *166*

10. Central Nervous System   169

- General Anesthetic Agents   *169*
- Sedatives and Hypnotics   *170*
- Anxiolytic Agents   *172*
- Antidepressants and Mood Stabilizers   *172*
- Antipsychotics   *173*
- Antiepileptics   *175*
- Opioid Analgesics   *176*

11. Integumentary System   181

- Antifungal Drugs   *181*
- Antiviral Drugs   *184*
- Drugs Used in the Treatment of Leprosy   *187*

12. Miscellaneous 189
- Emergency Medicines *189*
- Immunomodulators *195*
- Drug–Food and Drug–Drug Interactions *198*

Abbreviations   *201*

Bibliography   *207*

Index   *209*

CHAPTER 1

Basic Concepts

INTRODUCTION TO PHARMACOLOGY AND ITS TERMINOLOGY

- *Pharmacology*—It is a science of drugs; interaction of exogenously administered chemical molecules with specific molecules of living system which results in modulation of biologic function.
- *Pharmacokinetics*—What the body does to the drug.
- *Pharmacodynamics*—What the drug does to the body.
- *Drug*—Drug is any substance or product that is used or is intended to be used to modify or explore physiological systems or pathological states for the benefit of the recipient (WHO 1966).
- *Pharmacotherapeutics*—Application of pharmacodynamic information together with knowledge of the disease for its prevention, mitigation, and cure.
- *Clinical pharmacology*—Scientific study of drug in man; pharmacokinetic and pharmacodynamic investigation in healthy volunteers and in patients.
- *Chemotherapy*—Treatment of systemic infection and malignancy with specific drugs.
- *Pharmacy*—It is a science of compounding and dispensing drugs or preparing suitable forms for administration of drugs.
- *Toxicology*—Study of poisonous effects of drugs and other chemicals with an emphasis on detection, prevention, and treatment.
- *Drug nomenclature*—Three names. These are:
  1. *Chemical name*—It describes the substance chemically, e.g. para-aminophenol derivative.
  2. *Nonproprietary name*—This is accepted by competent scientific body; uniform; generic name, e.g. paracetamol (acetaminophen).
  3. *Brand name*—Name assigned by the manufacturing company; trade name, e.g. cetamol, panacet, cemol, cetanil.
- *Pharmacogenetics*—Drug responses that are governed by heredity.

- *Idiosyncrasy*—Inherited abnormal responses to drugs mediated by single gene; increased, deceased, and bizarre responses to drugs.
- *Pharmacovigilance*—Observation of safety, efficacy, and quality control of drug after it becomes available in the market.
- *Pharmacopeia*—An authorized book containing formulas and information that provide standard for preparation and dispensation of drugs.

DIFFERENT SOURCES OF DRUGS

- Synthetic
- Plant source
  - Alkaloids
  - Glycosides
  - Oils (essential oils, fixed oils, mineral oils)
  - Gums
  - Tannins
  - Resins
- Animal source
- Microbiological source
- Mineral source
- Genetically engineered drugs.

Synthetic

- Synthesized in the laboratory.
- Quality can be better controlled.
- Process is easier and cheaper.
- Chemical structure of prototype drug can be modified in search of better, safer, and more potent drug.
- For example, aspirin, paracetamol, phenytoin, chlorpromazine, amphetamine, etc.

Plant Sources

- Alkaloids
  - Nitrogenous heterocyclic bases derived from plants. For example atropine from *Atropa belladonna*, quinine from cinchona bark, morphine from *Papaver somniferum*, reserpine from *Rauwolfia serpentina,* and nicotine from tobacco leaves.
  - The names of all alkaloids usually end with "ne."

- Glycosides
  - Sugar-O-nonsugar (sugar portion → responsible for pharmacokinetic property, nonsugar → responsible for pharmacodynamic property).
  - Plant products in which sugar moiety is joined to nonsugar moiety with an ether linkage.
  - Sugar moiety → glucose = glucoside; sugar moiety → aminosugar = aminoglycoside.
  - For example, digoxin (*Digitalis purpurea*), ouabain (*Strophanthus gratus*), and aminoglycosides (*source: microorganisms*).
- Oils
  - Essential oils (or volatile oils)—Obtained from leaves or flower petals by steam distillation; steam volatile. Used as carminatives, astringent in mouthwashes, as a flavoring agent. For example, eucalyptus oil, clove oil, peppermint oil, etc.
  - Fixed oils—Nonvolatile. For example, groundnut oil, coconut oil, and olive oil.
  - Mineral oils—Mostly petroleum products; mainly used as vehicles for preparation of ointments. For example, hard and soft paraffin, as purgative-laxative, e.g. liquid paraffin.
- Gums
  - Colloidal exudates of plants. They either swell or dissolve or form adhesive mucilage in water.
  - It is used as emulsifying or suspending agents, e.g. gum acacia and gum tragacanth.
- Tannins
  - Nonnitrogenous phenolic derivatives from plant source.
  - It is used as astringent, e.g. tincture catechu.
- Resins—Polymers of volatile oil and are insoluble in water. For example, shellac (in enteric coating) and tolu balsam (as expectorant).

Animal Sources
- Hormones, vitamins, vaccines, sera.
- For example, insulin, vitamin B_{12}, thyroxin, etc.

Microbiological Sources
- Fungi—Penicillin, griseofulvin, cephalosporin.
- Bacteria—Polymyxin B, aztreonam, bacitracin, colistin.
- Actinomycetes—Aminoglycosides, macrolides, tetracycline, chloramphenicol.

Mineral Source
Ferrous sulfate (in anemia), magnesium sulfate (as purgative), aluminum hydroxide and sodium bicarbonate (as antacid), radioactive iodine I^{131} for the treatment of hyperthyroidism, etc.

Genetically Engineered Drugs (Fig. 1.1)
- Molecular biology, recombinant DNA technology, DNA alteration, gene splicing, etc.
- Hepatitis B vaccine, insulin.

DIFFERENT DOSAGE FORMS OF THE DRUGS
- Formulation—It is a recipe by which a drug is prepared. It contains the list of active ingredients and the other substances, like excipients, vehicles, flavoring agents, and preservatives, with the amounts contained therein.
- Dosage form—It is the form in which the formulation can be administered to the patient. For example, capsules, tablets, syrup, etc.
- Excipients—Pharmacologically inert substances which are added to the pharmaceutical preparation either to add bulk to the drug used in extremely small amount or to mask the unpleasant taste. For example, lactose, calcium lactate, starch, etc.
- Vehicle—Substance which is used to dissolve or suspend the drugs, in a pharmaceutical preparation. For example, gum acacia, petroleum jelly, etc.

Dosage forms can be classified as:
- Solid dosage forms:
  - Powders
  - Granules

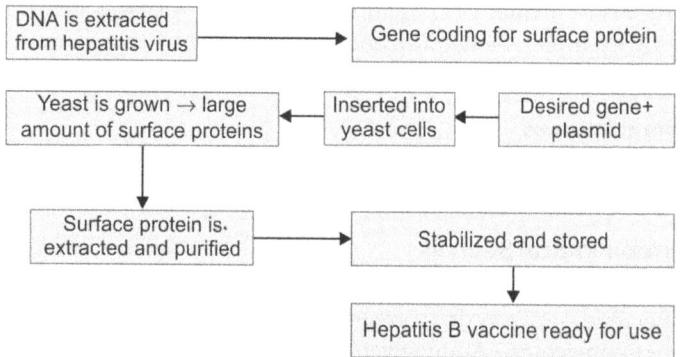

Fig. 1.1: Formation of genetically engineered hepatitis B vaccine.

Basic Concepts

- Tablets
  - Ordinary, sugar coated, film-coated, enteric coated, long (retard), pellets, lozenges, capsules
- Spansules.
- Liquid dosage forms:
  - Aqueous solutions
    - Syrup
    - Linctus
    - Injections
  - Aqueous suspensions
  - Mixtures and emulsions
  - Alcoholic solutions
    - Spirits
    - Elixir
- Drops—nasal/eye/ear drops
- Enema (liquid)—rectal
- Suppository (solid)—rectal
- Dosage forms for external uses:
  - Lotions
  - Liniments
  - Ointments
  - Paste
  - Gels
  - Aerosols
  - Suppositories
  - Transdermal adhesive patch
  - Ocusert.

IMPLEMENTATION OF PHARMACOLOGY IN NURSING PRACTICE

Solution—It is a dosage form of a medicine that contains solute in a solvent. It is of three types:

Percentage Solutions

- Weight in volume (W/V) solution—It means number of grams of the substance in 100 mL of the solution.
- Volume in volume (V/V) solutions—It means number of mL of the substance in 100 mL of the solution.
- Weight in weight (W/W) solution—It means number of grams of the substance in 100 g of the solution.

Basic Concepts

Molar Solutions
- One molar solution is obtained by dissolving one gram molecular weight of a substance in one liter of the solution.
- The quantity of the solid present in one molar solution is dependent on the volume of the solution. 100 mL of the solution contains 100 mmol of the solid and 10 mL will contain 10 mmol.

Solution Expressed in the Ratio
Solution may also be expressed as number of grams of solid in 1,000 mL. A 1 in 1,000 solution contains 1 g of the solid in 1,000 mL of the solution.

Exercises
- Calculate the quantity of sodium chloride present in 200 mL of half normal saline.
  Ans: 0.9 g.
  [Normal saline—0.9% NaCl; half normal—0.45% → 100 mL contains 0.45 g and 200 mL—0.9 g].
- Calculate the quantity of potassium permanganate present in 50 mL of potassium permanganate solution 1 in 1,000 and give instruction for preparing 1 in 10,000 solutions to be used as a gargle.
  Ans: 50 mg and water to be added is 450 mL.
  [1,000 mL contains 1 g (1,000 mg). So 50 mL contains 50 mg. Now, $N_1V_1 = N_2V_2$; $1/1,000 \times 50 = 1/10,000 \times V_2$; $V_2 = 500$ mL. So 450 mL should be added to the original solution. Hint—strength has been reduced by 10 times, so 10 times dilution is required, i.e. $50 \times 10 = 500$ mL, so 450 mL water should be added.]
- 0.5 mL of 1 in 1,000 solution of adrenaline is given subcutaneously in the treatment of an acute of asthma. What is the exact quantity of the adrenaline present in 0.5 mL?
  Ans: 0.5 mg.
  [100 mL solution contains 1 g (1,000 mg) adrenaline. So 0.5 mL → 0.5 mg].
- Calculate the amount of pilocarpine required to prepare 10 mL of 1% eye drops.
  Ans: 100 mg.
  [1% → 100 mL contains 1 g (1000 mg). So in 10 mL, 100 mg is required].

Basic Concepts

- How many mmol of sodium bicarbonate is there in 100 mL of 8.4% solution? (The molecular weight of sodium bicarbonate is 84).
  Ans: 100 mmol.
  [8.4% → 100 mL contains 8.4 g. Similarly, 1,000 mL contains 84 g. Note 84 is the mol wt of sodium bicarbonate. So this solution is in 1 M concentration. 100 mL contains 100 mmol (as 1,000 mL contains 1000 mmol)].
- If 1 mL of 1:200 solutions is diluted to 5 mL, what is the strength of resultant solution?
  Ans: 1: 1,000.
  [Note five times dilution, i.e. five times reduction in the strength or alternatively $N_1V_1 = N_2V_2$ can be applied].

ROUTES OF DRUG ADMINISTRATION

Factors affecting selection of route:
- Physical and chemical properties solid/gas/liquid/pH/solubility.
- Site of action.
- Effects of digestive juices/first pass metabolism.
- Rapidity of the response.
- Accuracy of the dosage.
- Condition of the patient.

Local Routes
- Topical **(Fig. 1.2)**
  - Skin: Ointment, cream, lotion, powder, spray.
  - Mucous membranes
    - Mouth/pharynx—Lozenges, mouthwashes, gargles
    - Eyes, ear, nose—Drops, ointments, nasal spray
    - Bronchi and lungs—Aerosols
    - Urethra—Jellys, bougies
    - Vagina—Pessaries, vaginal tablets
    - Anal canal—Suppositories.
- Deeper tissues
  - Intra-articular
  - Intrathecal.
- Arterial: Contrast media in angiography.
  Anticancer drugs in limb malignancies. In arterial routes, tourniquet is used to localize the drugs to the areas supplied by limb arteries.

Basic Concepts

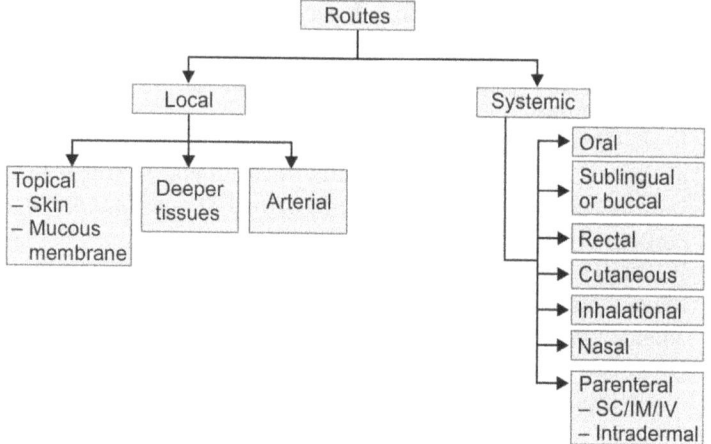

Fig. 1.2: Classification of different routes of drug administration.

Systemic Routes
- Oral
  - Advantages:
    - Most common, safer
    - More convenient, noninvasive
    - Painless.
  - Disadvantages:
    - Slow onset of action, first pass metabolism
    - Unpalatable drugs are difficult to take, gastric irritation
    - Uncooperative, unconscious, vomiting patients—oral route is not useful, e.g. tablets, capsules, syrups.
- Sublingual or buccal, e.g. nitroglycerine.
- Rectal, e.g. diazepam.
- Cutaneous: Transdermal therapeutic systems, e.g. insulin, testosterone, hyoscine, clonidine, etc.
- Inhalational, e.g. volatile liquids and gases.
- Nasal, e.g. desmopressin.
- Parenteral
  - Advantages:
    - Faster action, no gastric irritation
    - Unconscious patients
    - Liver is bypassed.

- Disadvantages:
  - Costlier, invasive, and painful
  - Self-administration is difficult
  - Local tissue injury.

Parenteral Routes
- Subcutaneous (SC)
- Intramuscular (IM)
- Intravenous (IV)
- Intradermal.

Main differences in local and systemic routes: Local routes—Direct application of the medicine, no/minimal systemic absorption, less side effects, safer route. Systemic routes—Drug reaches to the systemic circulation (hence the name systemic) and then only to the site of action, more side effects.

PRESCRIPTION WRITING AND COMMON ABBREVIATIONS
- ***Definition:*** A prescription is physician's written instructions to a pharmacist to supply drugs in a particular form to a patient. It includes directions to the pharmacist regarding the preparation and to the patient regarding the use of the medicament.
- The actual writing of a prescription order, if possible, should be done in the presence of the patient.
  This tends to impress upon the patient that the order is being written for his particular illness and increases his confidence in the physician.
- One should write without hesitation and with a degree of determination, concentration, and clarity indicative of the fact that the writer is perfectly acquainted with what he is doing.
- Erasing, crossing, and tearing of a prescription order in the presence of the patient and the poor procedure affects the patients psychologically and should be avoided.
- The prescription order should be laid aside for a few minutes, and then read before affixing one's signature.
- This is important because errors do occur, especially if talkative patients or relatives have distracted the physician.

A Prescription → Consists of Four Parts
1. Superscription
2. Inscription
3. Subscription
4. Signature.

Superscription
- Rx—Recipe, take thou
- The sign Rx is deemed to be an invocation to Jupiter—The God of healing.

Inscription
- Ingredients and the quantity
- The quantities of ingredients → should be in metric system.

Subscription
Directions to the dispenser as to the quantity to be dispensed.

Signature
- (Signature—let it be labeled) consists the directions to the patient. This part of the prescription declares:
  - The method of administration.
  - The dose (if the remedy is for internal use).
  - The time of administration or application.
  - The vehicle of administration or the means of application.
  - The part of the body to which the remedy is to be applied (if the remedy is for external use).
  - The patient's name, age, sex, and address; the particulars may be written at the top. Date should also be written at the top.
  - The prescriber's signature, name, and date.

Components of Prescription
- Physician and patient related
  - Doctor's name
  - Professional degree
  - Medical council registration number
  - Doctor's address and phone number
  - Patient's name
  - Patient's address
  - Diagnosis
  - The symbol Rx
  - Refill information
  - Prescriber's signature.
- Drug related
  - Dosage form
  - Appropriate drug
  - Strength of drug
  - Quantity to be dispensed
  - Direction for use.

Basic Concepts

Example for a prescription
Doctor's name: Dr. ABCD　　　　　　Academic degree: MD
Date: ....
• Medical Council Reg. No.　　　　Address/contact
• The patient's name: XYZ
Age/Sex: 25 yrs/M
Address: XXX
Diagnosis: Pharyngitis
• Superscription: Rx
• Inscription: Cap Amoxicillin 500 mg three times a day for 5 days
• Subscription: Dispense 15 capsules
• Take as instructed above after food, follow-up after 5 days
Signature

- The importance of giving clear written instructions to the patient or attendant regarding administration of drugs cannot be overlooked.
- The more the attention given to this, the more will be the patient's compliance with the treatment.

Some of the common Latin terms used in prescribing and dispensing are given below with their English equivalents.

Latin	Abbreviation	Meaning
• Recipe	Rx	Take thou
• Bis in die	bid (bd)	Twice a day
• Ter in die	tid (tds)	Thrice a day
• Quarter in die	qid	Four times a day
• Nocte	noct	At night
• Hora Somni	hs	At night
• Ante Cibos	ac	Before food
• Post Cibos	pc	After food
• Postprandial sugar	pps	Blood sugar after food
• Statim	Stat	Immediately
• Capsula	Caps	A capsule
• Si opus sit	sos	If needed
• Pro re nata	prn	As required
• Per oral	PO	By mouth

Contd...

Contd...

Latin	Abbreviation	Meaning
	D5W	Dextrose 5% in water
	IM	Intramuscular
	IV	Intravenous
	mg	Milligram
	OTC	Over the counter
	PR	Per rectum
	SC	Subcutaneous
	Sup	Suppository
	tab	Tablet
	tbsp	Tablespoon
	tsp	Teaspoon
	Vag	Vaginal
	q	Every

The following points should be followed while writing prescriptions:
- The same language should be used throughout preferably English.
- Each ingredient's name shall have a separate line.
- Each line begins with a capital.
- "Ditto" marks and "formulas" are not permissible.
- Be explicit in the directions given to the patient, as well as simple. No technical terms or abbreviations to be used here.
- Never sign a prescription or let it go out of your hands without carefully revising it.

PHARMACOKINETICS

Pharmacon—Drug, *kinesis*—movement; this is the study of *"what the body does to the drugs"*; study of movement of drug molecules inside the body.

Processes: ADME
- **A**bsorption
- **D**istribution
- **M**etabolism (biotransformation)
- **E**xcretion.

Absorption
Movement of drug from its site of administration into circulation.

Basic Concepts

Factors Affecting Absorption
- Aqueous solubility
- Concentration; ↑ concentration →↑ absorption
- Area of absorbing surface; ↑ area of absorbing surface → ↑ absorption
- Vascularity; ↑ vascularity →↑ absorption
- Route of administration:
  - Oral
  - SC/IM
  - Topical.
- Rate of absorption: IM (intramuscular) > SC (subcutaneous) > oral > topical.

Bioavailability
Fraction of administered dose of a drug that reaches the systemic circulation in the unchanged form.
- 100% for IV route
- <100% for other routes, due to following reasons:
  - Incomplete absorption
  - First pass metabolism
  - Local binding of a drug.

Bioequivalent—Two brand preparations of the same medicine having more or less same blood levels (bioavailability).

Biologically inequivalent—Two brand preparations of the same medicine having significantly different blood levels (bioavailability).

Chemically equivalent—Two brand products with the same amount of medicine. For example, two paracetamol preparations with 500 mg.

Therapeutic equivalence—Same clinical effects of different medicines of different therapeutic groups. For example, lowering of blood pressure by the same value with diuretics and beta blockers.

Distribution
Depends on:
- Lipid-solubility— ↑ solubility → more distribution.
- Ionization— ↑ ionization → less distribution.
- Plasma protein binding (PPB)—more PPB → less distribution.

Apparent Volume of Distribution
The volume that would accommodate all the drug in the body, if the concentration of a drug throughout the body was the same as in

plasma. Volume of distribution (Vd) is calculated as Vd = dose of drug administered/plasma concentration. The following considerations are important related to volume of distribution:
- Penetration into brain—Lipid-soluble medicines.
- Passage across placenta—Lipid-soluble medicines; at high concentration any drug can cross.
- Plasma protein binding (PPB)—More PPB, less volume of distribution.
- Tissue storage—Some drugs are deposited in tissues and have high volume of distribution:
  - Skeletal muscle/heart/kidney—Digoxin
  - Liver—Chloroquine
  - Retina—Chloroquine
  - Bone and teeth—Tetracycline
  - Adipose tissue—Thiopentone.

Metabolism (Biotransformation)
- Chemical alteration of the drug in the body.
- Lipid-soluble (nonpolar) drugs → lipid-insoluble (polar)—This is the main function or aim of drug biotransformation. Polar drug metabolites are easily excreted through kidney (due to ↓ tubular reabsorption).
- Metabolism may result in:
  - Inactivation
  - Activation of inactive drug—Known as prodrug, e.g. L-dopa (inactive) → dopamine (active) used in Parkinsonism.
- Two types of reactions:
  - **Phase I/nonsynthetic reactions**—Metabolites may be active or inactive. Examples—oxidation (by cytochrome P450 enzymes, almost 50–60% drugs are metabolized by this mechanism), reduction, hydrolysis, etc.
  - **Phase II/synthetic/conjugation reactions**—Metabolite is inactive. Examples—glucuronide conjugation (by UDP glucuronosyltransferase, major reaction in phase II), acetylation, glutathione and sulfate conjugation, etc.
- Metabolizing enzymes:
  - Microsomal—Cytochrome p450 enzymes, UDP glucuronosyltransferase.
  - Nonmicrosomal—Esterases, amidases, acetyltransferase, pseudocholinesterase.

- Enzyme induction—More synthesis of microsomal enzymes → faster drug metabolism → decreased efficacy. Examples of enzyme inducers—**St. John's Wort, A**nticonvulsants (phenytoin, carbamazepine), **B**arbiturates, **S**moking, Ethanol, **R**ifampin; Mnemonic—**St. John's Wort A**nd **B**arbiturates **S**timulate **E**nzyme **R**eaction (metabolism).
- Enzyme inhibition—Drug metabolism is inhibited → more chance of drug toxicity. Examples of enzyme inhibitors—**Grapefruit juice,** protease inhibitors (**I**ndinavir), **C**imetidine, **O**meprazole, **K**etoconazole, **E**rythromycin, **V**alproic acid/ **V**erapamil, **C**iprofloxacin; Mnemonic—**Grapefruit Juice I**nhibits **COKE V**ery mu**C**h.
- First pass metabolism—Metabolism of drugs in the gastrointestinal mucosa and/or liver on the way to systemic circulation after absorption—hence the name first pass as this is the first pass through hepatic tissues.
  Oral route— ↓ bioavailability (due to first pass metabolism)
  Liver disease— ↓ first pass metabolism.

Excretion
- Passage out of systemically absorbed drugs and their metabolites:
  - Urine, e.g. many drugs
  - Feces, e.g. erythromycin, oral contraceptives
  - Exhaled air, e.g. alcohol
  - Saliva and sweat, e.g. rifampin
  - Milk, e.g. alcohol, amoxicillin.
- Renal excretion:
  - Glomerular filtration
  - Tubular reabsorption
  - Tubular secretion.
  Renal excretion = (glomerular filtration + tubular secretion) - tubular reabsorption.
- Kinetics of elimination: Fundamental pharmacokinetic parameters are:
  - Bioavailability
  - Volume of distribution
  - Clearance.
- Clearance: It is the theoretical volume of plasma from which the drug is completely removed in unit time. Clearance = rate of elimination/plasma drug concentration.

- First-order kinetics: Rate of elimination is directly proportional to the drug concentration. Constant fraction of the drug is eliminated. Plasma half-life ($t^{1/2}$) and clearance are constant.
- Zero-order kinetics: Plasma half-life ($t^{1/2}$) and clearance are variable whereas rate of elimination is constant.
  Rate of elimination remains constant irrespective of drug concentration. A constant amount of the drug is eliminated.
- Plasma half-life (t½): It is time taken for the plasma concentration of a drug to be reduced to half of its original value. $t^{1/2} = 0.693 \times$ volume of distribution/clearance.
  For first-order kinetics, *4–5 plasma half-lives* are required for nearly complete elimination:
  - 1 t½—50% eliminated
  - 2 t½—75% (50 + 25) eliminated
  - 3 t½—87.5% (50 + 25 + 12.5) eliminated
  - 4 t½—93.75% (50 + 25 + 12.5 + 6.25) eliminated
  - 5 $t^{1/2}$—96.87% (50 + 25 + 12.5 + 6.25 + 3.12) eliminated.
- Loading dose: To attain therapeutic concentration. Loading dose = (volume of distribution × desired plasma drug concentration)/bioavailability
- Maintenance dose: To balance the rate of elimination.
  Maintenance dose = (clearance × steady-state plasma concentration × dosing interval)/bioavailability.

Steady-state Plasma Concentration (C^{ss}): Plateau Principle
- At steady state, rate of administration = rate of elimination (in = out).
- For the first-order kinetics, time to reach steady state only depends on the elimination half-life ($t^{1/2}$).
- When administered at intervals equivalent to half-life, a drug takes 4–5 half-lives to reach clinically acceptable steady state (though mathematically > 7 $t^{1/2}$ required).
- For drugs which follow first-order kinetics, *4–5 plasma half-lives* are required to achieve approximately 95% of C^{ss}, clinically acceptable steady state.
- When doses are repeated at the half-life interval, then
  After,
  1 $t^{1/2}$—50% of C^{ss} is achieved
  2 $t^{1/2}$—75% (50 + 25) of C^{ss} is achieved
  3 $t^{1/2}$—87.5% (50 + 25 + 12.5) of C^{ss} is achieved
  4 $t^{1/2}$—93.75% (50 + 25 + 12.5 + 6.25) of C^{ss} is achieved
  5 $t^{1/2}$—96.87% (50 + 25 + 12.5 + 6.25 + 3.12) of C^{ss} is achieved.

PHARMACODYNAMICS

Pharmacon—drug, *dynamics*—power; study of the power (effects, response) of drugs; this is the study of *"what drug does to the body"*. Mechanism of action, receptors, enzymes, agonism, antagonism, drug interactions, etc., come under pharmacodynamics.

Mechanism of Drug Actions

- Physical action
  - Mass of drug—Bulk laxatives
  - Adsorptive property—Charcoal
  - Osmotic activity—Mannitol
  - Radiopacity—Contrast media (barium sulfate).
- Chemical action—Antacids [e.g. $Al(OH)_3$] neutralize gastric HCl.
- Through enzymes—Stimulation: Adrenaline →↑ adenyl cyclase inhibition:
  - Nonspecific—Ethyl alcohol, phenol
  - Specific
    - Competitive—Physostigmine and neostigmine compete with acetylcholine for acetylcholine esterase.
    - Noncompetitive—Aspirin, indomethacin → cyclooxygenase.
- Through receptors
  - Receptor—It is a specific macromolecular component of the cell which binds and interacts with drug molecule.
  - Agonist—It activates receptor to produce an effect; brings about the conformational change.
  - Antagonist—It prevents the action of agonist on a receptor.
  - Inverse agonist—It activates a receptor to produce an effect opposite to that of agonist.
  - Partial agonist—It activates a receptor to produce submaximal effect.
  - Ligand—It is a drug molecule that binds to a receptor molecule.
  - Affinity—It is the ability of the drug to combine with a receptor.

Intrinsic Activity

- It is ability of drug to activate, i.e. to induce conformational change in the receptor after its binding to the receptor.
- Agonist-affinity + IA (IA = 1).
- Competitive antagonist-affinity; no intrinsic activity, IA = 0.
- Partial agonist-affinity + submaximal intrinsic activity (IA) (IA between 0.1 and 0.9).

- Inverse agonist-affinity + IA with minus sign [IA between 0 and (-1)].

Signal Transduction Mechanisms and Drug Action
- Amplification, integration, and transduction of drug receptor interaction as signal.
- Translation of receptor activation into functional response.

Five Major Mechanisms
1. G-protein coupled receptors (metabotropic):
   - Adenylyl cyclase or cAMP (cyclic adenosine monophosphate) pathway.
   - Phospholipase C or IP_3-DAG (inositol triphosphate-diacylglycerol) pathway.
   - Ion channel regulation (Na^+, K^+, Ca^{++}).
2. Receptors with intrinsic ion channels (ionotropic): Receptors enclose selective ion channels for Na^+, K^+, Ca^{++} or Cl^- e.g., cholinergic nicotinic receptors, $GABA_A$ receptor.
3. Enzymatic receptors—Receptor tyrosine kinase → insulin receptors.
4. JAK-STAT (Janus Kinase—Signal Transducer and Activator of Transcription) receptors: Binding to drug molecule → activation of JAK (Janus Kinase) → phosphorylation of STAT (Signal Transducer and Activator of Transcription) molecules → transcription; Examples—receptors for growth hormone, cytokines, etc.
5. Intracellular receptors: Receptors regulating gene expression—Steroid receptors.

   Receptor regulation: Upregulation (by antagonist), downregulation (by agonist), desensitization (by agonist).

Functions of Receptors
- To propagate regulatory signals
- To amplify the signal
- To integrate various extracellular and intracellular regulatory signals
- To help maintain the homeostasis.

Therapeutic Window Phenomenon
Optimal therapeutic effect is observed only in a narrow range of plasma drug log concentration, e.g. imipramine—50–150 ng/mL, clonidine—0.2–2 ng/mL.

Drug Potency and Efficacy

Drug Potency
It is the amount of drug to produce a response; relative, e.g. 10 mg morphine = 100 mg of pethidine.

Drug Efficacy
Maximum response that can be produced by a drug, e.g. morphine is more efficacious than aspirin.

Therapeutic Index
This is the measurement for safety of a drug, i.e. this gives the idea about how safe is the drug.

Therapeutic index (TI) = median lethal dose (LD_{50})/median effective dose (ED_{50}) ↑ TI → safer is the drug.

Therapeutic range → range between the dose which produces minimal therapeutic effect and the dose which produces acceptable adverse effects.

Drug Dose and Response Curve
It is the curve plotted against plasma drug log concentration and its clinical effects. It mainly helps to find out and compare potency, efficacy, and selectivity for different actions of many drugs **(Figs. 1.3 to 1.5)**.

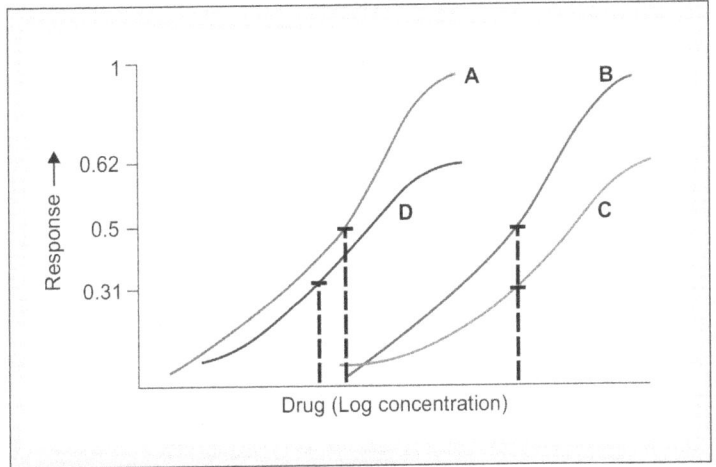

Fig. 1.3: Drug A (curve is more left) is more potent than drugs B and C. Drugs A and D are equipotent, but A is more efficacious than D (position of curve is the same, but peak is more for A than for D). Drugs A and B are equally efficacious (both have the same peaks).

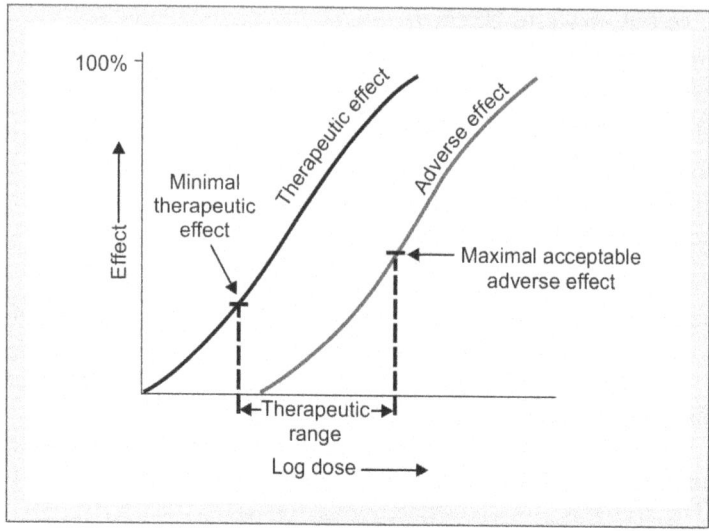

Fig. 1.4: Therapeutic range.

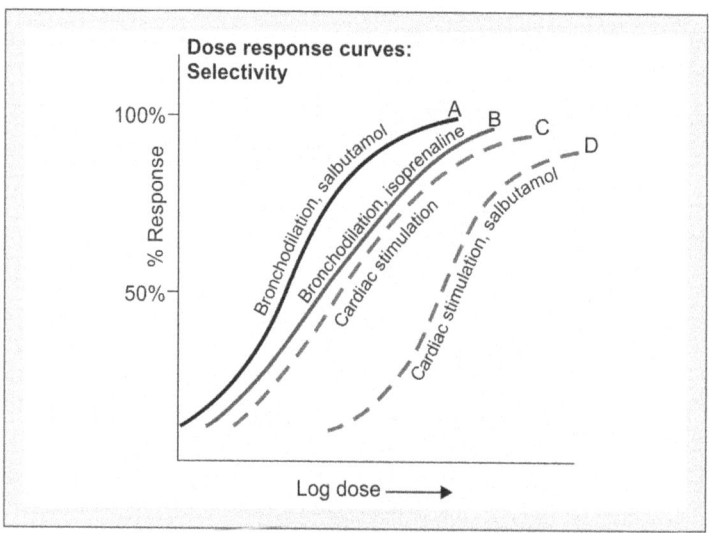

Fig. 1.5: Salbutamol is more selective for bronchodilation (curve A) than cardiac stimulation (curve D); isoprenaline shows bronchodilation and cardiac stimulation at the same dose (no selectivity for two effects because gap between curves B and C is very less).

Basic Concepts

Compare the height (in Y-axis) of drug dose and response curve (DRC) for the efficacy. ↑ Height → ↑ efficacy. For potency, compare the position (in Y-axis) of DRC. More toward the left → more potent is the drug.

Drug Interactions—Combined Effects of Drugs
- Synergism—Additive and supra-additive (potentiation).
- Antagonism—Physical, chemical, physiological (functional), receptor.

Synergism
Action of one drug is increased or facilitated by other drug:
- Additive—Effect of drugs A + B = effect of drug A + effect of drug B, e.g. aspirin + paracetamol.
- Supra-additive—Effect of drugs A + B > effect of drug A + effect of drugs B; effect of drugs A + B.

Antagonism
Action of one drug is inhibited by other:
Effect of drugs A + B < effect of drug A + effect of drug B
- Physical—For example, charcoal adsorbs alkaloids and prevents absorption (used in alkaloid poisoning).
- Chemical—Two drugs react and form an inactive product, e.g. $KMnO_4$ oxidizes alkaloids (used for gastric lavage in alkaloid poisoning) thiopentone sodium + succinylcholine.
- Physiological/functional—Different receptors/mechanisms → opposite effects on the same physiological effect, e.g. histamine and adrenaline on bronchial muscle and BP. Glucagon and insulin on blood sugar level.
- Receptor
  - Antagonist interferes with binding of agonist
  - Antagonist inhibits the action of agonist.

Competitive
The maximum response can be obtained by increasing the dose of agonist → surmountable antagonism, e.g. morphine and naloxone.

Noncompetitive
Maximum response cannot be obtained → insurmountable antagonism, e.g. diazepam and bicuculline.

Dose-response curves for competitive and noncompetitive antagonism are shown in Figures 1.6A and B.

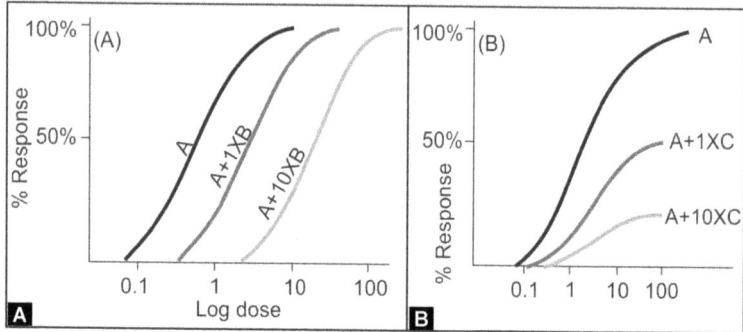

Figs. 1.6A and B: (A) Competitive antagonism (parallel rightward shift of DRC); (B) Noncompetitive antagonism [nonparallel rightward shift (flattening) of DRC]; A = agonist, B = competitive antagonist, and C = non-competitive antagonist.

FACTORS MODIFYING DRUG'S ACTION

- Body size: Individual dose = BW (kg)/70 × average adult dose
  Individual dose = BSA (m^2)/1.7 × average adult dose.
- Age
    Young's formula
    - Child dose = [age/(age + 12)] × adult dose
    Dilling's formula
    - Child dose = (age/20) × adult dose
    - Infant, adult, old: Multidrug therapy, liver and kidney status affects the doses of drugs.
- Sex
    - Ketoconazole, metoclopramide → gynecomastia
    - Pregnancy, menstruation, lactation
    - Female sex hormones, male sex hormones.
- Species and race: β-blockers are less effective in blacks.
- Genetics: Rates of drug metabolism; target organ sensitivity (four- to sixfold variation in doses), idiosyncrasy.
- Route of administration: MgSO$_4$, oral-purgative, local application-anti-inflammatory, IV—CNS depressant.
- Environmental factors and time of administration: Presence of food; morning administration of corticosteroids; exposure to insecticides, charcoal broiled meet, tobacco smoke.
- Psychological factor: Placebo—Inert substance which may produce response through psychological effect.

- Pathological states: Liver disease, kidney disease, heart disease.
- Tolerance
  - Natural
  - Acquired
  - Cross tolerance
  - Pharmacokinetic
  - Pharmacodynamic
  - Antimicrobial drug resistance.

ADVERSE DRUG REACTION

Types of Adverse Drug Reaction (Fig. 1.7)
- Side effects—Observed even with therapeutic dose
  - Mild and manageable.
- Secondary effects—Indirect consequences of main pharmacodynamic action
  - Superinfection by antibiotics
  - Weakening of host defense after glucocorticoids.
- Toxic effects—Exaggerated side effects and may occur due to
  - Overdose/prolong use
  - For example, heparin (bleeding), barbiturate (coma), sulfonamide (crystalluria/glomerulonephritis), gentamicin (nephrotoxicity).

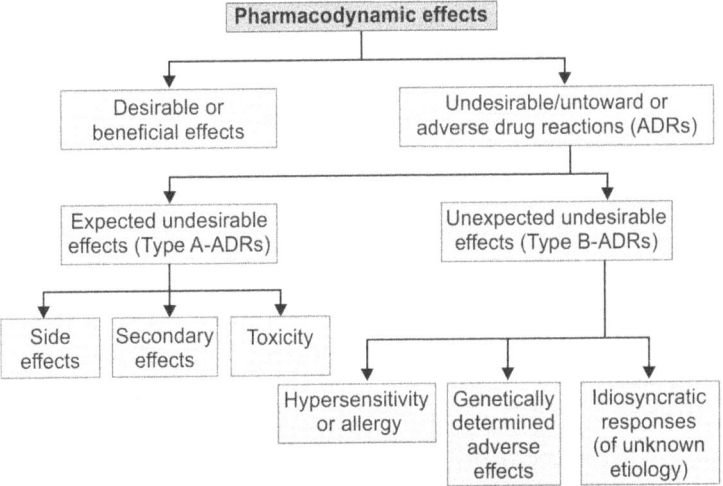

Fig. 1.7: Classification of pharmacodynamic effects of a drug.

Basic Concepts

Unexpected undesirable/type B adverse drug reaction (ADR):
- Arise unexpectedly, even in therapeutic dose
  - Immunological/pharmacogenetically mediated/idiosyncratic reaction.
- Types
  - Drug allergy—Resultant of the interaction of drug/metabolite/nondrug element
  - Genetically determined
  - G6PD deficiency
  - Atypical pseudocholinesterase.
- Idiosyncratic reaction.

Idiosyncratic Reactions and the Offending Drugs

Idiosyncratic reaction	Offending drugs
Hemolytic anemia, acute porphyria	Oxidizing agents, e.g. 8-aminoquinolines, sulfonamides
Malignant hyperthermia	A large number of CNS-active drugs and some antimicrobial agents
Hemolytic anemia, acute porphyria	Halothane, suxamethonium

Categories of drugs given by US-FDA based on fetal risk (teratogenicity)

	Risk category of drugs during pregnancy*	
Category		Examples
A No risk	Adequate studies in pregnant women have failed to demonstrate a risk to the fetus	Inj,. Mag. sulfate, thyroxine
B No evidence of risk in humans	Adequate human studies are lacking, but animal studies have failed to demonstrate a risk to the fetus or Adequate studies in pregnant women have failed to demonstrate a risk to the fetus, but animal studies have shown an adverse effect on the fetus	Penicillin V, amoxicillin, cefaclor, erythromycin, paracetamol, lidocaine
C Risk cannot be ruled out	No adequate studies in pregnant women, and animal studies are lacking or have shown an adverse effect on fetus, but potential benefit may warrant use of the drug in pregnant women despite potential risk	Morphine, codeine, atropine, corticosteroids, adrenaline, thiopentone, bupivacaine

Contd...

Contd...

Risk category of drugs during pregnancy*		
Category		Examples
D Benefit may outweigh potential risk	There is evidence of human fetal risk, but the potential benefits from use of the drug may be acceptable despite the potential risk	Aspirin, phenytoin, carbamazepine, valproate, lorazepam, methotrexate
X Contra-indicated	Studies in animals or humans have demonstrated fetal abnormalities. and potential risk clearly outweights possible benefit	Estrogens, isotretinoin, ergometrine thalidomide

* As per US-FDA

THERAPEUTIC DRUG MONITORING

It is measurement of serum drug concentration of medicaments to obtain optimal plasma drug concentration and benefit to the patient with minimal toxic adverse effects. For most drugs, therapeutic drug monitoring (TDM) is not necessary. TDM is important, if the drug has narrow therapeutic index (more toxic). Indications for TDM:
- To prevent the serious consequences of over or under dosing.
- To prevent the toxicity and to monitor the plasma concentration of the drugs having narrow therapeutic index.
- To prevent drug interactions.
- To check the patient compliance, especially in psychiatric patients.

Drugs which are Commonly Measured by TDM
- Cardioactive drug—Digoxin
- Antiseizure drugs—Phenytoin, phenobarbital, carbamazepine, ethosuximide, valproic acid
- Antibiotics—Amikacin, gentamicin, vancomycin
- Protease inhibitors—Indinavir, ritonavir
- Immunosuppressants—Cyclosporine, tacrolimus
- Tricyclic antidepressants—Amitriptyline
- Mood stabilizer—Lithium
- Bronchodilator—Theophylline.

Timing of specimen collection: This is the single most important factor in TDM. Steady-state concentration must be reached before

TDM begins (at steady state, rate of administration = rate of elimination). Generally, after five and half plasma half-lives steady-state is obtained. Blood sample is usually drawn at peak or trough state. Sample is taken at peak state for drugs given through IV route or if the patient has signs of toxicity shortly after use. However, for majority of drugs, the blood sample is drawn at trough, i.e. just before next dose.

Therapeutic Range (mg/L) of Drugs which are Commonly Monitored
- Digoxin—0.5-2.1
- Amiodarone—1-2.5
- Lignocaine—2-5
- Quinidine—2-5
- Flecainide—0.2-0.9
- Mexiletine—0.5-2.5
- Salicylates—150-300
- Theophylline—10-20
- Phenytoin—10-20
- Carbamazepine—5-12
- Sodium valproate—50-100
- Phenobarbitone—15-40
- Gentamicin, tobramycin, netilmicin—2-5
- Amikacin—5-15
- Vancomycin—10-440
- Lithium—0.6-1.2 mmol/L.

Information Required for Interpretations
- Time of blood sample collection in relation to last dose
- Duration of treatment with current dose
- Dosing schedule
- Age and gender of the patient
- Other drug therapy, if any
- Relevant disease states
- Reasons for the request, e.g. lack of effect, routine monitoring, susceptible toxicity, etc.

Therapeutic Drug Monitoring is not Required in the Following Conditions
- Drugs with high therapeutic index, e.g. vitamins, penicillins, cephalosporins, etc.

- Medicines with irreversible action or long duration of action (hit and run medicines)—MAO inhibitors, omeprazole, organophosphates, corticosteroids.
- Medicines with easily measurable clinical effects—Anti-hypertensives, diuretics, hypoglycemic, etc.
- In case of prodrugs—L-dopa.

ESSENTIAL DRUGS
- It can be defined as those drugs or medicines that satisfy healthcare needs of the majority of population; these should therefore be available at all times, inadequate amounts, and in appropriate dosage forms.
- It also known as essential medicines.
- Each country may have its own list depending upon the health care needs of the population.
- For example, paracetamol, amoxicillin, oral rehydration solution, antitubercular drugs, oral iron preparations, folic acid, oral contraceptive pills, etc.
- Pharmaceutical companies → "me-too drugs".
- Therapeutic "jungle."
- Only a handful of drugs → enough for most ailments.
- WHO published the first essential medicines list (EML) in 1977 and WHO updates the EML every two years; EML does not mean that the medicines outside it are not useful.

Criteria for Selection of Essential Drugs
- Should meet the needs of majority.
- Medicine must meet the prescribed standard of quality, bio-availability and shelf life.
- In case of more than one drug, priority should be given to that drug which has been thoroughly investigated.
- Most favorable pharmacokinetic data.
- Cost: Benefit ratio.
- Preferably a single drug compound.
- Should be in generic name.

Advantages
- Wider availability
- Substantial savings without affecting health care needs
- Improvement in drug dispensing and patient compliance
- Help planners and policy makers.

RATIONAL USE OF DRUGS

The Process of Rational Treatment
- Step 1: Define the patient's problem
- Step 2: Specify the therapeutic objective
  - What do you want to achieve with the treatment?
- Step 3: Verify the suitability of your P-treatment (P-drug)
  - Check effectiveness and safety (select P-drug based on **s**afety, **a**ffordability, **n**eed, **e**fficacy—**SANE**)
- Step 4: Start the treatment
- Step 5: Give information, instructions, and warnings
- Step 6: Monitor (and stop?) treatment.

Example: Patient 1
A 52-year-old taxi driver complains of a sore throat and cough which started two weeks earlier with a cold. He has stopped sneezing but still has a dry cough, especially at night. The patient is a heavy smoker who has often been advised to stop. Further history and examination reveal nothing special, apart from a throat inflammation. The doctor advises the patient to stop smoking, and writes a prescription for codeine tablets 15 mg, 1 tablet three times daily for 3 days.
1. Define the patient's problem: Sore throat and dry cough after a cold.
2. Specify therapeutic objective
   - Continuous irritation of the mucous membranes is the most likely cause of the cough.
   - The first therapeutic objective is therefore to stop this irritation by suppressing the cough, to enable the membranes to recover.
3. Verify the suitability of your P-treatment (P-drug)—apply the principles of SANE. Choose your P-treatment on the basis of efficacy, safety, suitability, and cost.
   - Need—Because of continuous exposure to traffic fumes and patient's habit of smoking, there is continuous irritation of pharyngeal mucosa. So this patient needs medication.
   - Codeine, noscapine, pholcodine, dextromethorphan.
   - Sedative antihistamines → diphenhydramine.
   - Codeine → P-drug for dry cough.
   - Adults → 30–60 mg 3–4 times daily.
4. Start the treatment
   - Rx
   - Tablet codeine 15 mg tid PO for 3 days, dispense 9 tablets.

5. Give information, instructions and warnings
   - It works within 2-3 hours.
   - It may cause constipation, and that it will make him sleepy if he takes too much of it or drinks any alcohol.
   - It should be advised to come back if the cough does not go within one week, or if unacceptable side effects occur.
   - Avoid alcohol, smoking, and traffic fumes.
6. Monitor (and stop?) treatment
   - If the patient does not return, he is probably better.
   - If there is no improvement and he does come back, there are three possible reasons:
     1. *The treatment was not effective.*
     2. *The treatment was not safe, e.g. because of unacceptable side effects.*
     3. *The treatment was not convenient.*
   - If the patient's symptoms continue, we will need to consider whether the diagnosis, treatment, adherence to treatment and the monitoring procedure were all correct.
   - In fact the whole process starts again.
   - Chronic diseases—Never-ending process.

DRUG INTERACTIONS

- *Beneficial*—Synergism is obtained. For example, paracetamol and ibuprofen combination in analgesia, aminoglycosides and penicillins in infective endocarditis, penicillins and probenecid in gram-positive bacterial infections.
- *Adverse*—Not wanted. Enzyme inducers may inhibit the efficacy of other medicines, when CNS depressants are used together → more CNS depression, when two nephro/ototoxic medicines are used → more toxicity, paracetamol + chronic alcoholism → hepatotoxicity.
- *Pharmacokinetic*—Interaction at the level of ADME.
  - Absorption—milk, antacids + iron → complex formation → less absorption.
  - Distribution—sulfonamides displace bilirubin in neonates → may cause kernicterus (unconjugated bilirubin easily crosses blood-brain barrier → deposition of bilirubin in brain tissues).
  - Metabolism—Enzyme inducers (rifampin, phenytoin, and carbamazepine inhibit the efficacy of oral contraceptive pills).

- Excretion—Penicillin and probenecid (probenecid inhibits the tubular secretion of penicillins and cephalosporins and prolongs duration of action).
- *Pharmacodynamic*—Interaction at the level of receptors. Alcohol + diazepam (Both these drugs are CNS depressants. So if taken together → greater degree of CNS depression, e.g. sedation).

CANCER CHEMOTHERAPY
Chemotherapy
- Chemotherapy for infections
- Cancer chemotherapy.

Depends on Three Main Factors
1. Type of cancer
2. Stage of cancer
3. Goal of the treatment
   - Curative
   - Palliative
   - Adjunctive.

Treatment Modality
- Chemotherapy
- Surgery
- Radiation therapy
- Hormonal therapy
- Combined modality approach/multimodality approach.

Types of Cancer Chemotherapy
- Primary induction chemotherapy: It is given as primary treatment approach for hematologic cancers and metastasized advanced solid tumors for which there is no other alternative.
- Adjuvant chemotherapy: It is given after surgical procedure or radiotherapy to kill the remaining malignant cells so as to have better prognosis and ↑ survival rate.
- Neoadjuvant chemotherapy: It is given before surgical procedure to shrink a tumor so as to have more effective surgical procedure.

Classification of Anticancer Drugs
- Cytotoxic drugs
  - Cell cycle specific
    - Antimetabolites: Methotrexate (folate antagonist); azathioprine, fludarabine, mercaptopurine (purine antagonist); cytarabine, fluorouracil (pyrimidine antagonist).

Basic Concepts

  - Antitumor antibiotics: Bleomycin, mitoxantrone.
  - Taxanes: Paclitaxel.
  - Vinca alkaloids: Vinblastine, vincristine.
  - Epipodophyllotoxin: Etoposide.
  - Camptothecin analog: Topotecan, irinotecan.
  – Cell cycle nonspecific
     - Alkylating agents: Cyclophosphamide, busulfan, carmustine.
     - Anthracyclines: Daunorubicin, doxorubicin.
  – Miscellaneous—Hydroxyurea, L-asparaginase, cisplatin, carboplatin.
- Drugs altering hormonal environment
  – Glucocorticoids—Prednisolone
  – Estrogen—Diethylstilbestrol
  – Antiestrogen—Tamoxifen
  – Antiandrogen—Flutamide
  – 5-α-reductase inhibitor—Finasteride.
- Tyrosine protein kinase inhibitor—Imatinib.
- Growth factor receptor inhibitor—Cetuximab.
- Aromatase inhibitor—Letrozole, anastrozole.
- Selective estrogen receptor downregulator—Fulvestrant.

Mechanism of Actions

Alkylating Agents
- Transfer alkyl group to cellular macromolecules, esp. DNA
- Cell cycle nonspecific (act on both dividing and resting cells).

Antimetabolites
Competitively inhibit utilization of normal substrate and get incorporated themselves producing dysfunctional macromolecules.

Vinca Alkaloids
- Mitotic inhibitors.
- Bind to microtubular protein—"tubulin" and prevent polymerization → failure of chromosomes to move apart during mitosis.

Antitumor Antibiotics
Break DNA strands and interfere with DNA function.

Taxane (Paclitaxel)
Enhances polymerization of tubulin → abnormal arrays/bundles of microtubules are produced.

Epipodophyllotoxins (Etoposide)
Inhibits DNA topoisomerase II.

Camptothecin Analogs (Topotecan and Irinotecan)
Inhibits DNA topoisomerase I.

Hormones
- Not cytotoxic.
- Modify the growth of hormone-dependent tumors.

Toxic Effects of Cytotoxic Anticancer Drugs
- Bone marrow
  - Neutropenia, lymphocytopenia—↑ infections
  - Thrombocytopenia—↑ bleeding tendency
  - Aplastic anemia—Fatigue, lethargy.
- Epithelial linings
  - Oral—Stomatitis, oral ulcers.
  - GIT—Gastric ulcers, bleeding, nausea, and vomiting.
  - Skin—Alopecia, dermatitis.
- Reproductive function
  - Oligozoospermia—Male infertility.
  - ↓ Ovulation, amenorrhea—Female infertility.
- Pregnancy
  - Abortion/fetal death.
  - Teratogenesis.
- Carcinogenicity: Secondary cancers (leukemia, lymphomas).
- Hyperuricemia: Gout (due to ↑ cell destruction →↑ purine metabolism →↑ uric acid).
- Neurotoxicity: Peripheral neuropathies, e.g. cisplatin.
- Nephrotoxicity: Cisplatin, ifosfamide, and methotrexate.
- Hemorrhagic cystitis: Cyclophosphamide and ifosfamide (acrolin-toxic metabolite causes bladder irritation and damage → bleeding episodes); mesna—for protection.
- Hepatotoxicity
  - Asparaginase, cytarabine, mercaptopurine, thioguanine, and methotrexate.
  - Jaundice, hepatitis, and elevation of liver transaminase enzymes.
- Cardiotoxicity
  - Daunorubicin and doxorubicin.
  - Dexrazoxane—Cardioprotectant and is given with the above drugs.

Basic Concepts

- Hypersensitivity reactions: Asparaginase, carboplatin, cisplatin.
- Tumor lysis syndrome
  - In leukemias and lymphomas, due to spontaneous lysis and release of intracellular content such as K^+, PO^4, and uric acid.
  - Preventive measures—Adequate hydration, alkalinization of urine and administration of allopurinol (uric acid synthesis inhibitor), and/or rasburicase and pegloticase (uricase preparations → break down uric acid into allantoin).

Methods to Reduce Toxicity

- Toxicity blocking drugs
  - Folinic acid (a form of tetrahydrofolate) or leucovorin or citrovorum factor ↓ toxicity (bone marrow depression and hepatotoxicity) of methotrexate
  - Ondansetron—↓ nausea and vomiting caused mainly by alkylating agents
  - Dexrazoxane—↓ cardiotoxicity of daunorubicin and doxorubicin
  - Mesna (2-mercaptoethane sulfonate Na)—↓ toxicity (hemorrhagic cystitis) of cyclophosphamide and ifosfamide
- Control of hyperuricemia
  - Allopurinol (uric acid synthesis inhibitor), and/or rasburicase and pegloticase (uricase preparations → break down uric acid into allantoin), alkalinization, plenty of fluids.
- Pulse therapy: Gap of 2-3 weeks interval → normal cells recover; malignant cells recover more slowly.
- Topical administration of anticancer drugs as far as possible: Skin, buccal mucosa, vagina.
- Platelet/granulocyte transfusion.
- Bone marrow transplantation.

ANTIMICROBIAL AGENTS (AMAs) AND BASIC PRINCIPLES OF ANTIMICROBIAL CHEMOTHERAPY

Antibiotics

Substances produced by micro-organisms which inhibit/kill other micro-organism at very low concentrations.

Antimicrobial Agents

Both natural and synthetic compounds that inhibit/kill micro-organisms.

Classifications

Chemical Structure
- Sulfonamides and related drugs—Sulfadiazine, dapsone
- Diaminopyrimidine—Trimethoprim, pyrimethamine
- Quinolone—Nalidixic acid, ofloxacin, ciprofloxacin
- β-lactam antibiotics—Penicillins, cephalosporins
- Tetracycline—Oxytetracycline, doxycycline
- Nitrobenzene derivative—Chloramphenicol
- Aminoglycosides—Streptomycin, gentamicin
- Macrolides—Erythromycin
- Nitroimidazole—Metronidazole
- Polyene derivatives—Amphotericin B
- Imidazole derivatives—Ketoconazole, miconazole.

Mechanism of Actions
- Cell wall synthesis inhibitors—Penicillin, cephalosporins, cycloserine, vancomycin
- Leakage from cell membrane—Polymyxin, amphotericin B
- Protein synthesis inhibitors—Tetracyclines, chloramphenicol, erythromycin
- Misreading of mRNA code and affecting permeability—Aminoglycosides
- DNA gyrase inhibitors—Fluoroquinolones
- Interfere with DNA function—Metronidazole
- DNA synthesis inhibitors—Acyclovir, zidovudine
- Interfere intermediary metabolism—Sulfonamides.

Type of Organism Against which Primarily Active
- Antibacterial—Penicillins, aminoglycoside
- Antifungal—Ketoconazole, itraconazole
- Antiviral—Zidovudine, acyclovir
- Antiprotozoal—Chloroquine, metronidazole
- Anthelmintic—Mebendazole, pyrantel, niclosamide.

Spectrum of Activity
- Narrow spectrum—Penicillin G, streptomycin
- Broad spectrum—Tetracycline, chloramphenicol.

Types of Actions
- Bacteriostatic—Sulfonamides, tetracycline, chloramphenicol
- Bactericidal—Penicillin, aminoglycosides.

Antibiotics Obtained From
- Fungi—Penicillin, cephalosporin
- Bacteria—Polymyxin B, colistin
- Actinomycetes—Aminoglycoside, macrolides, tetracyclines.

Problems with Use of AMAs
- Toxicity—Gastric irritation, diarrhea, ototoxicity, nephrotoxicity
- Hypersensitivity reactions
- Drug resistance
- Superinfections (suprainfections)—Broad spectrum antibiotics; Candida, *Clostridium difficile* (clindamycin, tetracycline, etc.)
- Nutritional deficiency: Vitamin B complex, vitamin K.
- Masking of an infection: Single dose of penicillin to cure gonorrhea (may mask syphilis).

Principles of Antimicrobial Chemotherapy
Patient-related Factors
- Age—Tetracycline (children)—Tooth discoloration, chloramphenicol (in newborn)—Gray baby syndrome; sulfonamides kernicterus; aminoglycosides—Deafness.
- Renal and hepatic function
   - Renal failure—Aminoglycoside, cephalosporin, vancomycin, amphotericin B
   - Hepatic disease—Erythromycin estolate, pyrazinamide, tetracycline, etc.
- Local factors—Pus, anaerobic environment
- Drug allergy
- Pregnancy
- Breastfeeding
- Genetic factors—G6PD deficient-hemolysis, primaquine, sulfonamides, etc.
- Impaired host defense.

Organism-related Factor
Clinical diagnosis.

Drug Factors
- Spectrum of activity
- Type of activity
- Relative toxicity
- Route of administration
- Evidence of clinical efficacy
- Cost.

SULFONAMIDES AND COTRIMOXAZOLE (FOLATE ANTAGONISTS) AND QUINOLONES AND FLUOROQUINOLOES (DNA SYNTHESIS INHIBITORS)

Sulfonamides
- First antimicrobial agents
- Domagk—Prontosil.

Chemistry
- Derivatives of sulfanilamide (para-amino-benzene sulfonamide).
- Sulfonamide N—Solubility, potency and pharmacokinetic property.
- Free amino group in para (N_4) position → antibacterial activity.

Classifications
- Short acting (4–8 h): Sulfadiazine.
- Intermediate acting (8–12 h): Sulfamethoxypyrazine, sulfamoxole.
- Long acting (approximately 7 days): Sulfadoxine, sulfamethoxypyrazine.
- Special purpose sulfonamide: Sulfacetamide sodium, sulfasalazine, mafenide, silver sulfadiazine.

Antibacterial Spectrum
- Primarily bacteriostatic against gram-positive and gram-negative organisms.
- *Streptococcus pyogenes, Haemophilus influenzae, H. ducreyi, Calymmatobacterium granulomatis, Vibrio cholerae.*
- *Chlamydia, Actinomyces, Nocardia, Toxoplasma.*

Mechanism of Action
Woods and Fildes (1940)—Sulfonamide being structural analog of PABA inhibits bacterial folate synthetase → folic acid is not formed.

Evidence in Favor
- PABA—Antagonizes the effect
- Only those microbes synthesizing PABA are susceptible
- Pus—Purine, thymidine, and PABA—Decrease the action.

Resistance
Gonococci, pneumococci, *Staphylococcus aureus*, meningococci, *E. coli, Shigella*.

Resistant Mutant May
- Produce increased amounts of PABA
- Decreased affinity for folate synthetase
- Adopt an alternative pathways in folate metabolism.

Pharmacokinetics
- Rapid and complete absorption from GIT
- PPB (10-95%)
- Widely distributed, cross BBB, and placenta
- Metabolism → in liver, nonmicrosomal, acetylation at N_4
- Excretion—Glomerular filtration, less soluble in acidic urine → crystalluria.

Adverse Drug Reaction
Relatively Common
- Nausea, vomiting, epigastric pain
- Crystalluria
- Hypersensitivity reactions
- Hepatitis
- Topical use is not permitted → contact dermatitis; ocular use is permitted
- Hemolysis in G6PD deficiency
- Kernicterus.

Interaction
It may displace phenytoin, tolbutamide, warfarin, methotrexate from protein binding → toxicity may occur.

Uses
- Systemic therapy as monotherapy—Rare now.
- Suppressive therapy—Chronic UTI, streptococcal pharyngitis.
- Combined with trimethoprim, sulfamethoxazole—*P. carinii* and nocardiosis.
- Combined with pyrimethamine, sulfadoxine—Malaria.
- Sulfacetamide sodium—Ocular preparation.
- Topical silver sulfadiazine or mafenide—It is used to prevent infection on burn dressing.

Cotrimoxazole
Trimethoprim + sulfamethoxazole → cotrimoxazole (1969).

Trimethoprim
- Diaminopyrimidine related to antimalarial drug—Selectively inhibits bacterial dihydrofolate reductase (DHFRase)
- > 50,000 times higher affinity for bacterial DHFRase
- Wide distribution, crosses BBB and placenta
- Partly metabolized in liver excreted in urine.

Combinations
- Sequential block in folate metabolism—Bactericidal.
- Both have t½ ~10 h; optimal synergism in most bacteria; MIC of each agent may be reduced by 3-6 times.
- Dose ratio 1:5 (trimethoprim: sulfamethoxazole).
- Plasma concentration ratio 1:20.
- Resistance—Slow to develop compared to either drug; mostly through mutational or plasmid mediated acquisition of a DHFRase having low affinity.

Adverse Drug Reactions
- Nausea, vomiting, stomatitis.
- Folate deficiency—Megaloblastic anemia.
- Patient with renal disease—Uremia.
- In AIDS patients with *Pneumocystis carinii* infection—Bone marrow depression.
- Elderly—Bone marrow depression.

Uses
Cotrimoxazole
- UTI
- RTI (both upper and lower)
- Typhoid
- Bacterial diarrhea and dysentery
- Chancroid
- Granuloma inguinale
- *Pneumocystis carinii.*

Trimethoprim
- UTI
- Prostatitis.

Quinolones
- Synthetic compounds.
- Primarily active against gram-negative bacteria.
- Newer fluorinated compounds—Also inhibits gram-positive bacteria.
- Nalidixic acid (1960).
- Fluorinated compounds—High potency, expanded spectrum, slow development of resistance, better tissue penetration, and good tolerability.

Nalidixic Acid
- Active against *E. coli*, Proteus, Klebsiella, *Enterobacter, Shigella* but not pseudomonas
- Inhibits bacterial DNA gyrase—Bactericidal
- Resistance develops rapidly
- High concentration in urine (20–50 times higher than plasma) → lethal to common urinary pathogens.

Adverse Drug Reaction
Relatively Infrequent
- GI upset and rashes
- Neurological toxicity—Vertigo, visual disturbances, seizures
- Parkinsonism like symptoms
- Phototoxicity
- G6PD deficiency—Hemolysis.

Uses
- As urinary antiseptic (nitrofurantoin should not be used with nalidixic acid concurrently—antagonism may occur).
- In diarrhea by Proteus, *E. coli, Shigella*, Salmonella (especially in ampicillin resistant *Shigella* enteritis).

Fluoroquinolones
Quinolone antimicrobials having one or more fluorine substitutions.

Classifications
- First generation (1 fluoro substitution in 1980s).
- Norfloxacin, ciprofloxacin, ofloxacin, pefloxacin.
- Second generation (2 fluoro substitutions in 1990s).
- Lomefloxacin, sparfloxacin, levofloxacin, gatifloxacin, moxifloxacin.

Mechanism of Actions
- Inhibit DNA gyrase (two subunits A and B; A-nicking and resealing of DNA, B-introducing negative supercoiling); have higher affinity for A subunit.
- Recent studies → gram-positive bacteria → topoisomerase IV which nicks and separates daughter nuclei strands after DNA replication; greater affinity of fluoroquinolones for this enzyme → higher potency against gram-positive organism.

Mechanism of Resistances
- Chromosomal mutation producing a DNA gyrase or topoisomerase IV with reduced affinity for FQs.
- Reduced permeability or increased efflux mechanism of these drugs across bacterial membranes.

Ciprofloxacin (Prototype)
- Most potent first generation agent.
- Most susceptible organisms → gram-negative bacilli including Enterobacteriaceae and *Neisseria*.

Pharmacokinetics
- Rapidly absorbed from GIT, food delays the absorption.
- High tissue penetrability → high concentration in lung, sputum, muscle, bone, prostate, and phagocytes.
- Excreted primarily in urine, both by glomerular filtration and tubular secretion; urinary and biliary concentration is 10-50 times higher than in plasma.

Adverse Drug Reactions
- Good safety; 10% patients; withdrawal in 1.5%.
- Gastrointestinal—Nausea, vomiting, anorexia, bad taste.
- CNS—Dizziness, headache, anxiety, impairment of concentration and dexterity.
- Skin/hypersensitivity.
- Tendonitis and tendon rupture.

Interactions
- ↑ Levels of theophylline, caffeine, and warfarin by ciprofloxacin → toxicity may occur.
- NSAID may enhance the CNS toxicity.
- Antacids, sucralfate, and iron salts reduce gastric absorption.

Uses
- UTI—Both uncomplicated and complicated (3 days regimen)
- Gonorrhea—Single 500 mg dose (~100% cure)
- Chancroid—500 mg BD for 3 days
- Bacterial gastroenteritis
- Typhoid—Ciprofloxacin is the drug of choice; 500-750 mg BD for 10 days; for typhoid carriers 750 mg for 2-4 weeks
- Bone, soft tissues, and gynecological and wound infections
- Respiratory tract infections—Not the primary drug
- Tuberculosis in combination therapy

- Gram-negative septicemia
- Meningitis
- Conjunctivitis by gram-negative bacteria.

CELL WALL SYNTHESIS INHIBITORS—PENICILLIN, CEPHALOSPORIN, AND VANCOMYCIN

Penicillin
- β-lactam antibiotic.
- First discovered by Alexander Fleming in 1929.
- First used clinically in 1941.
  Antibacterial spectrum: Gram-positive bacteria mainly; extended spectrum: Also effective against gram-negative and anaerobes.
- Other β-lactam compounds are:
  - Cephalosporins
  - Carbapenems
  - Monobactams.

Mechanism of Actions
- Interferes with bacterial cell wall synthesis
- Transpeptidase enzyme is inhibited
- Penicillin binding proteins (PBPs) in the bacteria are the target receptors for penicillins
- Cell wall deficient structures that swell and burst → bacterial lysis.

Classifications
- Penicillins (PnG).
- Acid-resistant penicillin (PnV).
- Penicillinase-resistant penicillins:
  - Nafcillin
  - Cloxacillin
  - Methicillin
  - Dicloxacillin.
- Extended spectrum penicillins:
  - Aminopenicillins—Ampicillin, amoxicillin, bacampicillin.
  - Carboxypenicillins—Carbenicillin, ticarcillin.
  - Ureidopenicillins—Piperacillin, mezlocillin.
  - Mecillinam.

Bacterial resistance:
- Due to one of the four general mechanisms:
  - Inactivation by penicillinase/β-lactamase.
  - Modification of target PBPs.

- Impaired penetration of drug to target PBPs (located deeper under lipoprotein barrier).
- The presence of an efflux pump.

Adverse Effects
- Local irritancy and direct toxicity:
  - Pain at IM injection site
  - Nausea on oral ingestion
  - Thrombophlebitis of injected vein
  - Bleeding.
- Hypersensitivity (1-10%):
  - Anaphylaxis—Rare (1-4/10,000)
  - Prevention—History, scratch test or intradermal test.
- Superinfections
- Jarisch-Herxheimer reaction:
  - Penicillin injected in syphilitic patient may produce fever, chills, and myalgia
  - Sudden release of spirochetal lytic products.

Uses of Penicillin G
- Streptococcal infections (SABE—Subacute bacterial endocarditis)
- Pneumococcal infections
- Meningococcal infections
- Syphilis
- Diphtheria
- Tetanus and gas gangrene
- Prophylactic uses:
  - Rheumatic fever
  - Gonorrhea or syphilis
  - Bacterial endocarditis
  - Surgical infections.

Uses of Amoxicillin
- UTI, RTI, meningitis, gonorrhea
- Typhoid
- Bacillary dysentery—*Shigella*
- Cholecystitis
- SABE
- Septicemia and mixed infections.

Adverse drug reactions—Diarrhea, incomplete absorption, and rashes.

Cephalosporins

Mechanism of Action

Bind to cephalosporin binding proteins → inhibition of transpeptidation process → formation of imperfect cell wall → lysis of bacteria (bactericidal).

Antibacterial spectrum: Many gram-positive (mainly first and second generation cephalosporins), negative bacteria and beta lactamase producing bacteria (third, fourth, and fifth generations). Cephalosporins are not effective against **LAME** [**L**isteria *monocytogenes*, **A**typicals (e.g. Chlamydia, *Mycoplasma*), **M**RSA (methicillin-resistant *Staphylococcus aureus*), and **E**nterococci].

Classifications

Classified as:
- First generation (1960s)
- Second generation (1970s)
- Third generation (1980s)
- Fourth generation (1997–1998)
- Fifth generation (after 1998).

First-generation Cephalosporins
- Oral: Cephalexin, cefadroxil, cephradine.
- Parenteral: Cefazolin, cephalothin, cefadroxil.

Uses
- UTI
- Staphylococcal infections (cellulitis or soft tissue abscess)
- Cefazolin—It is the drug of choice in surgical prophylaxis (because of better tissue penetration).

Second-generation Cephalosporins
- Oral: Cefaclor, cefuroxime axetil.
- Parenteral: Cefuroxime, cefotetan, cefamandole, cefoxitin.
- Peritonitis (cefoxitin and cefotetan—more active against anaerobes).
- Respiratory tract infections (cefaclor—more active than first generation).
- Community acquired pneumonia.
- Gonorrhea (PPNG)—Single dose IM.
- Meningitis.

Third-generation Cephalosporins
- Oral: Cefixime, cefpodoxime proxetil, cefdinir, ceftibuten.
- Parenteral: Ceftriaxone, cefotaxime, ceftazidime, ceftizoxime, moxalactam.

Uses
- Ceftriaxone
  - Meningitis
  - Gonorrhea and chancroid
  - Community acquired pneumonia
  - Complicated UTIs, abdominal sepsis, septicemia
  - Multidrug-resistant typhoid fever.

Fourth-generation Cephalosporins
Parenteral: Cefpirome and cefepime.

Fifth-generation Cephalosporin
Ceftaroline (can bind mutated penicillin binding proteins in MRSA).

Adverse Effects
- Hypersensitivity reactions—Fever, skin rash, eosinophilia, angioedema.
- Cross sensitivity with penicillins.
- Superinfection—Pseudomembranous colitis and diarrhea (third generation).
- Bleeding—Cefamandole, cefoperazone, cefotetan (hypoprothrombinemia and destruction of vitamin K producing colonic bacteria).
- Local irritation after IM injection.

Vancomycin
- Inhibits gram-positive bacterial cell wall synthesis by complexing with D-alanyl-D-alanine portion of the terminal end of peptidoglycan pentapeptide.

Uses
- MRSA infections.
- Orally in pseudomembranous colitis (if metronidazole is ineffective); IV route only.

Adverse Drug Reaction
Red neck syndrome—Chills, fever, intense flushing (due to histamine release), ototoxicity, nephrotoxicity, eosinophilia.

PROTEIN SYNTHESIS INHIBITORS—TETRACYCLINE, CHLORAMPHENICOL, AMINOGLYCOSIDES, AND MACROLIDES

Tetracyclines

Classifications
- Group I—Tetracycline, chlortetracycline
- Group II—Demeclocycline, methacycline
- Group III—Doxycycline, minocycline.

Mechanism of Action
Inhibit protein synthesis by binding to 30S ribosomes.

Adverse Drug Reactions
- Epigastric pain, nausea, vomiting, diarrhea
- Liver damage
- Kidney damage
- Phototoxicity
- Discoloration of teeth (if used during pregnancy or in childhood)
- Hypersensitivity reactions
- Superinfection (pseudomembranous colitis).

Precautions and Contraindications
- Pregnancy, during lactation, and in children
- Renal disease, hepatitis.

Uses
- Venereal diseases—Lymphogranuloma venereum, granuloma inguinale
- Atypical pneumonia by *Mycoplasma pneumoniae*
- Cholera
- Brucellosis
- Plague
- Relapsing fever/rickettsial infections.

Chloramphenicol

Mechanism of Action
- Binds with 50S ribosome → inhibits protein synthesis
- High dose → inhibits mammalian protein synthesis.

  Bone marrow suppression.

Adverse Drug Reactions
- Bone marrow suppression: Aplastic anemia, agranulocytosis, thrombocytopenia, pancytopenia.
- Hypersensitivity reaction: Rashes, fever.
- Irritative effects: Nausea, vomiting, diarrhea.
- Superinfections.
- Gray baby syndrome
    - Baby stops feeding, becomes hypnotic and hypothermic; vomiting, distended abdomen, irregular respiration, grayish appearance.
    - Due to inability of newborn to metabolize and excrete chloramphenicol.

Uses
- Enteric fever: Ciprofloxacin, ceftriaxone, cotrimoxazole, ampicillin/amoxicillin
- *H. influenzae* meningitis
- Anaerobic infection—*Bacteroides fragilis*
- Intraocular infections
- Brucellosis, cholera, and rickettsial and chlamydial infections.

Aminoglycosides
Drugs
Systemic Agents
- Streptomycin
- Gentamicin
- Kanamycin
- Tobramycin
- Amikacin.

Local Agents
- Neomycin
- Framycetin.

Properties
- Highly water-soluble; highly ionized
- Not absorbed when given orally
- Bactericidal
- Active in alkaline medium; interfere with bacterial protein synthesis
- Narrow margin of safety
- Primarily active against aerobic gram-negative bacilli.

Mechanism of Actions
- Bactericidal
- Streptomycin binds to 30S ribosome, but other agents also bind to additional site on 50S ribosome and 30S–50S interface as well.

Drug Resistance
- Synthesis of drug inactivating enzymes
- Mutation of ribosomal proteins
- Reduced efficiency of transport mechanism.

Toxic Effects
- Ototoxicity
- Nephrotoxicity
- Neuromuscular blockade.

Precautions and Interactions
- Pregnancy—Contraindication (ototoxicity)
- Avoid concurrent use of other ototoxic and nephrotoxic drugs
- Old age; kidney diseases
- Use of muscle relaxants
- Do not mix with other drugs in the same syringe or infusion bottle.

Uses
Streptomycin
- Tuberculosis
- Subacute bacterial endocarditis
- Plague
- Tularemia.

Gentamicin
- Respiratory infections
- *Pseudomonas*, *Proteus* or *Klebsiella* infections, burns, UTI, middle ear infections, septicemia
- Meningitis (by gram-negative bacteria)
- Subacute bacterial endocarditis.

Neomycin
- Topically: Infected wound, ulcers, burns.
- Orally for
  - Preparation of bowel surgery
  - Hepatic coma.

Macrolides

Drugs
- Erythromycin
- Roxithromycin
- Clarithromycin
- Azithromycin.

Mechanism of Actions
- Inhibits bacterial protein synthesis by binding to 50S ribosome
- Mostly gram-positive and few gram-negative bacteria are inhibited
- Static at low concentration and cidal at higher concentration.

Adverse Drug Reactions
Erythromycin
- Gastrointestinal—Epigastric pain, diarrhea
- Reversible hearing impairment (at high dose)
- Hypersensitivity reactions—Rashes
- Hepatitis with cholestatic jaundice (resembling viral hepatitis—Erythromycin estolate).

Uses
As a First Choice Drug
- Atypical pneumonia by mycoplasma
- Whooping cough
- Chancroid.

As an Alternative to Penicillin
- Streptococcal pharyngitis, tonsillitis, and most respiratory infections
- Diphtheria
- Syphilis and gonorrhea.

As a Second Choice Drug
- Campylobacter enteritis
- Legionnaires' pneumonia
- *Chlamydia trachomatis*
- Penicillin-resistant staphylococcal infections.

Newer drugs—Roxithromycin, clarithromycin, and azithromycin
Similar to erythromycin except
- Newer drugs are more potent, effective, and safer.
- These have longer duration of action and less gastric irritation.

ANTISEPTICS AND DISINFECTANTS

- Disinfectants are those chemical substances which are used to destroy or inhibit the growth of pathogenic vegetative bacteria (not their spores) on inanimate (nonliving) surfaces such as glass wares or surgical instruments.
- For example, formaldehyde, phenols, ethyl alcohol, soaps, etc.
- Antiseptics are those chemical substances which are used to destroy pathogenic bacteria (not the spores) on animate surfaces such as skin and mucous membranes.
- Chlorhexidine, listerine, povidone iodine, etc.
- Differences between disinfectants and antiseptics seem to be small and overlapping.
- Some antiseptics in higher concentration may work as disinfectants.
- Similarly, some disinfectants in lower concentration may serve as antiseptics.
- Sterilization—It is a process of killing all living organisms including spores, viruses, and fungi.
- Germicide—Antiseptic and disinfectant.

A Good Antiseptic/Disinfectant should be

- Chemically stable.
- Cheap.
- Nonstaining with acceptable color and odor.
- Cidal not only static.
- Active against all pathogens—Bacteria, fungi, viruses and protozoa.
- Able to spread through organic films.
- Active even in the presence of blood, pus exudates, and excreta.

Classification

Which Act by Precipitating (Coagulating) Bacterial Proteins

- Aldehyde—Formaldehyde, glutaraldehyde
- Phenols—Phenol in 57% ethanol, cresol, triclosan
- Alcohol—Ethyl alcohol, isopropyl alcohol
- Heavy metal salts—Silver nitrate, zinc-calamine lotion.

Which Act by Complexing with Sulfhydryl (sh) Group of Bacterial Enzymes

Mercurial antiseptics—Mercurochrome, nitromersol.

Which Act by Oxidizing the Sulfhydryl (sh) Groups of Bacterial Enzymes
- Chlorophores—Chlorine dioxide, sodium hypochlorite
- Iodophores—Povidone iodine, tincture iodine
- Oxidizing agents—Hydrogen peroxide, potassium permanganate.

Which Alter Properties of Bacterial Cell Wall
Chlorhexidine, cetylpyridinium chloride, benzalkonium chloride.

Ectoparasiticides
Topical Route
- Against lice (*Pediculus*) and mite (*Sarcoptes/Acarus scabiei*)
- Permethrin—Drug of choice
- Lindane (gamma benzene hexachloride, BHC)
- Benzyl benzoate—Contraindicated in children
- Crotamiton—Second choice; may be preferred in child.

Oral Route
Ivermectin—This is only drug which can be administered via oral route.

COMMON POISONS AND ANTIDOTES
Poisoning is the state produced by introduction of a poison into the body. Symptoms of poisoning vary widely from agent to agent. Specific treatment of poisoning depends upon the type of the poisoning agent. However, some general principles are presented here:

General Measures
- *To prevent further exposure or absorption of the poison:* Remove the victim from the poisoning source. Sometimes, contaminated clothing has to be removed (in case of organophosphorus poisoning) and contaminated skin should be washed with soap and water thoroughly. The patient should be moved to the fresh air. Except in corrosive poisoning, the patient is made to vomit to prevent further absorption. Some adsorbents like activated charcoal, tannic acid, and magnesium oxide can be administered. In some heavy metal poisoning, chelating agents can be administered through nasogastric tube to help prevent the further absorption.
- *To increase the rate of elimination:* Forced diuresis is carried out. Sometimes either alkalinization or acidification of urine may also help increase the excretion of poison depending upon the type of agent.

Supportive Measures

These are adopted to maintain the airway, breathing, and circulation (ABC). Airway should be checked and cleaned if any obstruction is present. Respiration, blood pressure, and heart rate should be checked. Oxygen inhalation, fluid and electrolyte balance, proper maintenance, and monitoring of blood pressure should be carried out at regular intervals.

Specific Antidotes

In case known poisoning by the known agent and if the antidote or antagonist is available, it is administered as soon as possible to reverse the toxic effects. For example, the followings are some specific antidotes:
- Organophosphorus poisoning—Atropine
- Morphine poisoning—Naloxone
- Benzodiazepine—Flumazenil
- Atropine (belladonna poisoning)—Physostigmine

Early type of mushroom poisoning/muscarine type/cholinergic type—Atropine.

Other Measures

If the situation is not improving from the above measures and if there is still some hope for the recovery by filtering out the poisonous agent, hemodialysis can be performed.

CHELATING AGENTS

- Dimercaprol
- Dimercaptosuccinic acid (succimer)
- Disodium edetate
- Calcium disodium edetate
- Penicillamine
- Desferrioxamine
- Deferiprone.

Dimercaprol (BAL—British Anti-Lewisite)

- Oily, pungent smelling viscous liquid
- It is used in As, Hg, Bi, Ni, and Cu poisonings
- SH group binds with the metals
- Contraindication in Fe and Cd poisoning
- IM route.

Dimercaptosuccinic acid (succimer)
- Similar to BAL
- Water-soluble, orally effective
- In As, Hg, and Pb poisonings
- Disodium edetate (Na_2EDTA)
  - Potent chelator of calcium
  - Slow IV infusion
  - In hypercalcemia.

Calcium disodium edetate (CaNa2EDTA)
- In Pb, Zn, Cd, Mn, Cu, radioactive materials
- Ionized
- IV (IM is painful).

Penicillamine
- Degradation product of penicillin
- Strong Cu chelation (Wilson's disease–1956)
- In Cu, Hg, Pb, Zn
- D-isomer
- Orally before (1 h) or after food (2 h).

Desferrioxamine (Deferoxamine)
- Ferrioxamine → Iron containing, actinomycetes
- Fe removal → desferrioxamine → high affinity for Fe (1g → 85 mg elemental Fe)
- Acute iron poisoning
- Parenteral route.

Deferiprone (Deferasirox)
- Orally active iron chelator.

Drug Overdose and Poisoning and Specific Antidotes

Drug or compound	Antidote
Organophosphates, carbamates (insecticides, pesticides, war gases)	Atropine (receptor antagonist), also pralidoxime in organophosphate poisoning (pralidoxime-acetylcholine esterase reactivator)
Morphine and other opioids	Naloxone (IV), naltrexone (oral)
Benzodiazepines (e.g. diazepam, alprazolam)	Flumazenil
Atropine (belladonna or Datura poisoning)	Physostigmine

Contd...

Contd...

Drug or compound	Antidote
Early type of mushroom poisoning (presentation within 1 h of ingestion and cholinergic features)	Atropine (in delayed types of mushroom poisoning, atropine is contraindicated)
Paracetamol (acetaminophen)	N-acetylcysteine (it replenishes glutathione)
β-blockers	Glucagon
Amphetamines	NH_4Cl (acidifies urine → ↑ excretion)
Carbon monoxide	100% O_2 (hyperbaric O_2)
Digoxin	Anti-dig Fab (digoxin immune Fab, Digibind)
Aspirin	$NaHCO_3$ (alkalinizes urine → ↑ ↑excretion)
Tricyclic antidepressants (TCAs)	$NaHCO_3$ (alkalinizes plasma → ↑ binding of TCAs to cardiac Na+ channels)
Warfarin	Vitamin K (delayed effect), fresh frozen plasma (immediate effect)
Streptokinase, urokinase	Aminocaproic acid
Cyanide	Nitrite + thiosulfate or hydroxocobalamin
Heparin	Protamine sulfate (chemical antagonist)
Copper, arsenic, gold	Penicillamine
Mercury, arsenic, gold	Dimercaprol (BAL), succimer (oral)
Methanol, ethylene glycol (antifreeze)	Fomepizole, ethanol (ethyl alcohol)
Methemoglobin	Methylene blue, vitamin C
Neostigmine, physostigmine	Atropine
Iron	Deferoxamine/Deferoxamine (parenteral—IV/IM/SC), Deferasirox/Deferiprone (oral)

VITAMINS, VACCINES AND ANTISERA

Vitamins

Classifications

Fat-soluble vitamins—Vitamins A, D, E, and K may cause cumulative toxicity. Water-soluble vitamins—Vitamin B complex, C—not stored, no/minimal toxicity.

Vitamin A

Actions

Visual cycle—opsin + 11-cis retinal (vitamin A) → Rhodopsin—dim light → opsin + all transretinal (this breakdown of rhodopsin generates visual nerve impulse and a person is capable of dark adaptation, can see in dim light. So in deficiency state, rhodopsin synthesis is compromised and a person may suffer from night blindness).

Epithelium—Proliferation, ↑ mucous secretion, ↓ keratinization (vitamin A ointment can be used as keratinolytic in hyperkeratinized condition).

Reproductive and immunological function—Vitamin A is required for proper functioning.

Deficiency
- Dryness of eye (xerosis)
- Bitot's spot—Triangular shiny gray spots in conjunctiva
- Keratomalacia—Softening of cornea
- Night blindness—Complete blindness (due to permanent damage to the rods)
- Phrynoderma—Dry rough skin with papules
- Hyperkeratinization
- Infertility
- Growth retardation.

Uses
- As prophylaxis
- Treatment of deficient state
- In skin diseases—Acne, psoriasis, ichthyosis.

Vitamin E

Actions

Antioxidant—It prevents oxidative damage to the cells and biological membranes (other antioxidants—β-carotene, vitamin C, cysteine, methionine, selenium, and chromenols).

Deficiency state—No specific condition.

Use

As an antioxidant agent.

Vitamin D and K

Vitamin D and K have been explained in their respective sections—Endocrine and blood section (See Calcification and Bone Turnover:

Basic Concepts

Parathormone, vitamin D and Calcitonin for vitamin D, page no. 141, and Drugs Affecting Coagulation and Bleeding for vitamin K, page no. 64).

Water-soluble vitamins are vitamin B complex and vitamin C.

Thiamine (Vitamin B_1, Aneurine)

Actions
Active form—Thiamine pyrophosphate acts as a coenzyme in carbohydrate metabolism, decarboxylation of ketoacids, and hexose monophosphate shunt (synthetic thiamine antagonists—Pyrithiamine and oxythiamine).

Deficiency
- Dry beriberi—Neurological symptoms (main features)—Polyneuritis, numbness, muscular weakness, "wrist drop," "foot drop," paralysis of limbs.
- Wet beriberi—Cardiovascular symptoms (main features)—Palpitation, breathlessness, CHF, anasarca (whole body edema).

Uses
- As prophylaxis
- In beriberi
- In acute alcoholic intoxication—It is given with glucose, also in chronic alcoholism to treat Wernicke's encephalopathy and Korsakoff's psychosis
- In neurological and cardiovascular disorders.

Niacin (Vitamin B_3)

Niacin—Nicotinic acid and nicotinamide.

Actions
Nicotinic acid → nicotinamide → it is a component of NAD (nicotinamide adenine dinucleotide) its phosphate NADP → involved in oxidation-reduction reactions.

Nicotinic acid → vasodilator and hypolipidemic agent, can be used in peripheral vascular disease and in hyperlipidemia.

Deficiency
Pellagra—Disease of 3 Ds—Dermatitis (sunburn like), diarrhea, and dementia (with hallucinations and insomnia).

Uses
- In prophylaxis.
- Treatment of pellagra.

- In Hartnup's disease (tryptophan transport is impaired) and carcinoid syndrome (tryptophan is used to produce 5-HT)- niacin supplement (inside the body tryptophan is converted into nicotinic acid, 60 mg tryptophan = 1 mg nicotinic acid).

Pyridoxine (Vitamin B_6)
- Active form—Pyridoxal phosphate—Coenzyme for transaminases and decarboxylases.
- Antitubercular drug isoniazid inhibits the generation of pyridoxal phosphate may produce pyridoxine deficiency → peripheral neuritis.
- Hydralazine, cycloserine, and penicillamine interfere with pyridoxine utilization → deficiency state.

Deficiency
- Peripheral neuritis
- Seborrheic dermatitis
- Glossitis
- Confusion
- Growth retardation
- Decrease in seizure threshold.

Uses
- Prophylaxis in alcoholics, with isoniazid therapy.
- In drug-induced deficiency state (isoniazid, hydralazine, cycloserine and penicillamine).

(Vitamin B_{12} has been dealt in blood section. So please refer to the Hematinics used in anemia).

Vitamin C (Ascorbic Acid)

Actions
- Antioxidant.
- Involved in hydroxylation of proline and lysine residues of protocollagen → required for formation and stabilization of collagen triple helix (so, in vitamin C deficiency, there is inherent collagen defect →↑ capillary fragility → more prone to hemorrhage and decreased wound healing).
- Conversion of folic acid → folinic acid.
- Biosynthesis of adrenal steroids, catecholamines, oxytocin, and vasopressin.

Deficiency
Scurvy—Swollen and bleeding gums, subcutaneous and subperiosteal hemorrhages, growth retardation, anemia.

Uses
- Prophylaxis
- Treatment of scurvy
- Postoperatively to enhance wound healing
- In anemia increases iron absorption
- To acidify urine.

Vaccines and Antisera

Vaccines and antisera → enhance body's immunity power.

Vaccines (contain antigens—either whole organism or part of it, live or killed or attenuated) are involved in active immunity (body produces antibodies), prophylactic.

Antisera and immunoglobulins impart passive immunity (already formed antibodies are injected to the body), curative.

Vaccines, antisera, and immunoglobulins have potential risk of anaphylaxis. So adrenaline (1:1,000), glucocorticoids, and antihistamines should be in hand before administration.

Classification of Vaccines

Killed Vaccines (Inactivated)

Bacterial
- Typhoid-paratyphoid
- Cholera
- Whooping cough (pertussis)
- Meningococcal
- Plague
- *Haemophilus influenzae* type b.

Viral
- Poliomyelitis inactivated (IPV, Salk)
- Rabies
- Influenza
- Hepatitis A and B.

Live Attenuated Vaccines

Bacterial
Bacillus Calmette-Guérin (BCG).

Viral
- Poliomyelitis oral alive (OPV, Sabin)
- Mumps
- Measles
- Rubella
- Varicella.

Toxoids—Bacterial Exotoxins with Antigenicity
- Tetanus
- Diphtheria.

Combined Vaccines
- DPT—Diphtheria-pertussis-tetanus
- MMR—Measles-mumps-rubella
- DPT + hepatitis B + *Haemophilus influenzae* type b
- DT-DA—Double antigen → precipitated toxoids of tetanus + diphtheria.

Immunization Schedule (Also, Please Refer to the Government's Recent Guidelines on Immunization Schedule of Our Country)

Time of administration	Name of vaccine
At birth	BCG + OPV (first dose) + hepatitis B (after 12–24 h)
At 6 weeks	DPT + OPV + hepatitis B
At 10, 14 weeks	DPT + OPV
At 6 months	Hepatitis B
At 9 months	Measles
At 15–18 months	DPT + MMR + OPV (booster dose)
At 4–5 years	DT-DA + OPV (booster dose), Typhoid-paratyphoid
At 10 years	TT
At 16 years	TT
For pregnant females	
At 16–24 weeks of pregnancy	TT (first dose)
At 24–34 weeks of pregnancy	TT (second dose)

Antisera and Immunoglobulins

Antisera—Purified horse serum with specific antibodies, high risk of anaphylaxis.

Immunoglobulins—Purified human gammaglobulins → nonspecific or specific (hyperimmune) against an antigen, low risk of anaphylaxis.

Horse Antisera
- Tetanus antitoxin—Prophylaxis when nonimmunized person gets highly contaminated and risky wounds with high risk of tetanus, human globulin is preferred.
- Gas gangrene antitoxin given for the prophylaxis and therapy of gas gangrene.
- Diphtheria antitoxin given in clinical diphtheria.
- Antirabies serum given in suspected exposure along with rabies vaccine.
- Antisnake venom polyvalent given to neutralize Cobra venom, Russell's viper venom, saw-scaled viper venom, and krait venom.

Human Immunoglobulins
- Normal human gammaglobulin prophylaxis for hepatitis A and B, measles, mumps, and poliomyelitis.
- Anti-D immunoglobulin human IgG against Rh (D), used for prevention of postpartum/postabortion formation of antibodies in Rho (D) negative women → prevents Rh hemolytic disease in future offspring.
- Tetanus immunoglobulin is given for prophylaxis when nonimmunized person gets highly contaminated and risky wounds with high risk of tetanus.
- Rabies immunoglobulin given in suspected exposure along with rabies vaccine.
- Hepatitis B immunoglobulin given in persons exposed to hepatitis B positive blood or blood products.

Note: If anaphylaxis occurs, adrenaline (1:1,000), glucocorticoids, and antihistamines should be given.

CHAPTER 2

Blood

HEMATINICS USED IN ANEMIA

Iron, vitamin B_{12} and folic acid.

Fe Preparation and Doses

Oral

- Ferrous sulfate—20-30% Fe → 200 mg tab
- Ferrous gluconate—22% Fe → 300 mg tab
- Ferrous fumarate—33% Fe → 200 mg tab
- Colloidal ferric hydroxide—50% Fe → 200/400 mg tab
  - The elemental Fe content should be considered/dose.
  - 200 mg elemental Fe/day → maximum hematopoietic response, a rise in hemoglobin level by 0.5-1 mg/dL per week after iron therapy is an indicator for good response to iron therapy.
  - 30 mg/day → prophylactic dose.

Adverse Drug Reactions

- Gastric irritation—Nausea, vomiting, epigastric pain
- Constipation
- Metallic taste, staining of teeth.

Parenteral

- Iron-dextran (colloidal solution → 50 mg Fe/mL → IM/IV)
- Iron-sorbitol-citric acid complex → 50 mg Fe/mL only IM.

Adverse Drug Reactions

- Pain at the site of IM injection, pigmentation of skin
- Fever, headache, palpitation, dyspnea.

Uses

- Fe deficiency anemia
- Prophylaxis—It is used in menstruating females, pregnancy, acute blood loss, chronic diseases, and menorrhagia
- Megaloblastic anemia.

Vitamin B$_{12}$

Preparation and Doses
- Cyanocobalamin
- Hydroxocobalamin
- Pernicious anemia → IM/SC, hydroxocobalamin is preferred
- Other deficiency → 10-30 μg/day; oral
- Prophylaxis → 3-10 μg/day; oral.

Uses
- Treatment of megaloblastic anemia
- Other vitamin B$_{12}$ deficiency states
- As prophylaxis.

Adverse Drug Reactions
- Safe even in high dose
- Anaphylaxis on IV injection (rare).

Folic Acid

Preparation and Doses
- Folic acid—5 mg tab oral/injection; therapeutic dose—2-5 mg/day; prophylactic dose—0.5 mg/day.
- Folinic acid—Injection 3 mg/mL; this is 5-formyl-THFA; need not be reduced by DHFRase.

Uses
- Megaloblastic anemia
- As prophylaxis
- Methotrexate toxicity.
  Folinic acid—Leucovorin/citrovorum factor.

Adverse Drug Reaction
Nontoxic.

ANTIMALARIAL DRUGS

Classification Based on the Plasmodial State

Schizonticides
These kill the schizonts of the malarial parasite:
- Tissue (hepatic) schizonticides:
  - Primary tissue schizonticides—Act on preerythrocytic state, e.g. proguanil, pyrimethamine, and primaquine.
  - Secondary tissue schizonticides—Act on exoerythrocytic state, e.g. primaquine.

- Blood schizonticides—Prevent erythrocytic schizogony to terminate attack of malarial fever:
  - Fast-acting high efficacy—Chloroquine, mepacrine, mefloquine, halofantrine, artemisinin, and atovaquone.
  - Slow-acting low efficacy—Pyrimethamine, proguanil, sulfonamides.

Gametocides
Destroy the gametes or make them ineffective in the host's blood so that mosquito cannot transmit the disease, e.g. primaquine—For all four species of plasmodium.

Chloroquine and quinine—All four except *P. falciparum*.

Different Forms of Antimalarial Therapies
- Causal prophylaxis:
  - Preerythrocytic stage; proguanil, primaquine.
  - Primaquine 0.5 mg/kg/day (check G6PD level because primaquine administration in G6PD deficient individuals causes hemolysis, due to decreased NADPH production → oxidized glutathione can't be regenerated to a reduced form, and primaquine causes oxidative damage to RBCs → hemolysis)
- Suppressive prophylaxis:
  - Schizonticides—Suppress erythrocytic phase and prevent attacks of malarial fever; chloroquine, proguanil, mefloquine, doxycycline.
  - Chloroquine 300 mg/week.
- Clinical cure:
  - Erythrocytic schizonticides to terminate the episodes; blood schizonticides.
  - Chloroquine 600 mg followed by 300 mg after 8 h and 300 mg/day for next 2 days.
  - Pyrimethamine 25 mg + sulfadoxine 500 mg tab—three tabs single dose (chloroquine resistant).
  - Artemisinin-based combination therapy (ACT).
- Radical cure: Exoerythrocytic stage; primaquine 15 mg/day for 14 days.
- Suppressive cure: Radical cure followed by suppressive therapy; chloroquine 300 mg/week for 10 weeks.
- Gametocidal:
  - To clear gametes from patient's blood: It increases transmission
  - Primaquine 45 mg single dose after clinical cure.

Artemisinin-based Combination Therapy (ACT)—Oral Therapy
Advantages of ACT Rapid Clinical Cure and Parasite's Clearance
- Cure rates are high → 95% and low relapse (recrudescence)
- Better side effect profile.
- No development of resistance.

ACT Regimens (WHO Approved Regimens)
- Artesunate + mefloquine → artesunate 100 mg BD for 3 days and mefloquine 750 mg on 2nd days and 500 mg on 3rd days
- Artemether + lumefantrine → artemether 80 mg BD and lumefantrine 480 mg BD for 3 days
- Artesunate and sulfadoxine + pyrimethamine → artesunate 100 mg BD for 3 days and sulfadoxine 1,500 mg + pyrimethamine 75 mg single dose
- Dihydroartemisinin (DHA) + piperaquine (PPQ) → DHA 120 mg and PPQ 960 mg daily for 3 days
- Artesunate + amodiaquine → artesunate 200 mg and amodiaquine 600 mg once a day for 3 days.

DRUGS FOR VISCERAL LEISHMANIASIS (KALA-AZAR) AND FILARIASIS

Drugs for Leishmaniasis
Antimonials—Contain Antimony Metal, Sb.
Sodium stibogluconate—Used by intramuscular route (meglumine antimoniate in French-speaking countries).

Others
- Amphotericin B—Highly efficacious, used by intravenous route
- Miltefosine—Developed in India, given orally, teratogenic—contraindicated in pregnancy
- Paromomycin—Intramuscular route
- Allopurinol—Weak effect
- Ketoconazole—Weak effect.

Diamidine—Outdated
Pentamidine.

Drugs for Filariasis (*Wuchereria Bancrofti, Brugia Malayi*)
- Diethyl carbamazepine (DEC) citrate—It is the drug of choice
- Ivermectin
- Albendazole.

DRUGS AFFECTING COAGULATION AND BLEEDING

Classification of Drugs used in Coagulation and Thromboembolic Disorders
- Coagulants
- Anticoagulants
- Fibrinolytics
- Antifibrinolytics
- Antiplatelet drugs.

Coagulants
- Vitamin K: Vitamin K_1 (plant)—Phytonadione; K_2 (bacteria)—Menaquinones; K_3 (synthetic)
  - Fat-soluble—Menadione
  - Water-soluble—Menadione sodium bisulfite; menadione sodium diphosphate.
- Miscellaneous
  - Fibrinogen
  - Antihemophilic factor
  - Adrenochrome
  - Monosemicarbazone
  - Rutin, ethamsylate
  - Desmopressin.

Vitamin K

Mechanism of Action

It acts as a cofactor for the synthesis of coagulation factors II, VII, IX, and X.

Preparations
- Phytonadione—10 mg/mL IM injection
- Menadione—0.66 mg cap
- Menadione sodium bisulfite—20 mg tab.

Uses

For prophylaxis and treatment of clotting factor deficiency
- Dietary deficiency of vitamin K
- Prolonged antimicrobial therapy
- Obstructive jaundice
- Newborns [vitamin K_3 hemolysis (G6PD deficiency, competes for glucuronide conjugation with bilirubin → kernicterus; contraindicated; phytonadione is the drug of choice)]

- Uses of rutin and ethamsylate
  - Menorrhagia
  - After abortion
  - Hematuria
  - Postpartum hemorrhage
  - Epistaxis
  - Melena
  - After tooth extraction.

Anticoagulants

Used in Vitro
- Heparin
- Calcium complexing agents: Sodium citrate, sodium oxalate, sodium edetate.

Used in Vivo
- Heparin—low molecular weight heparin
- Oral anticoagulants:
  - Coumarin derivatives—Bishydroxycoumarin (dicumarol), warfarin sodium, acenocoumarol
  - Indandione derivative—Phenindione.

Mechanism of Action of Heparin
Combines with antithrombin III → activation of antithrombin III → inactivation of factor Xa and IIa.

Dosage
- 5,00–10,000 U IV (high dose)
- 500 U SC (low dose)
- aPTT 1.5–2.5 times normal value
- Clotting time—2 times.

Side Effects
- Bleeding
- Thrombocytopenia
- Transient and reversible alopecia
- Hypersensitivity reactions.

Contraindications
- Bleeding disorders
- Thrombocytopenia
- Severe hypertension, piles, peptic ulcer
- Subacute bacterial endocarditis

- Ocular and neurosurgery, lumbar puncture
- Chronic alcoholics, liver cirrhosis, renal failure.

Low Molecular Weight Heparins (Fractionated Heparins)—MW 3000–7000
- Examples: Enoxaparin, reviparin.
- Uses
  - Prophylaxis of deep vein thrombosis and pulmonary embolism in high-risk patients (undergoing surgery, stroke, immobilized patients).
  - Treatment of deep vein thrombosis.
  - Unstable angina.
  - To maintain patency of cannulae and shunts in dialysis patients.

Heparin antagonist—Protamine sulfate.

Oral Anticoagulants

Warfarin

Mechanism of Actions

- Inhibits the synthesis of vitamin K-dependent clotting factors (II, VII, IX, and X).
- Available in 1, 2 and 5 mg tab.

Uses

- Deep vein thrombosis and pulmonary embolism
- Myocardial infarction
- Unstable angina
- Rheumatic heart disease and atrial fibrillation
- Vascular surgery, prosthetic heart valves, hemodialysis.

Side Effects

- Bleeding (ecchymosis, epistaxis, hematuria, GI bleeding, internal hemorrhages)
- Alopecia
- Dermatitis
- Diarrhea.

Dose Regulation

Prothrombin time
- 2–2.5—Prophylaxis of DVT
- 2–3—Treatment of DVT, pulmonary embolism, TIAs
- 3–4.5—Recurrent thromboembolism, MI, prosthetic heart valves.

Contraindications
Pregnancy—Fetal warfarin syndrome → hypoplasia of nose, eye socket, hand bones, and growth retardation.

Fibrinolytic (Thrombolytic) Agents
- Streptokinase
- Urokinase
- Alteplase (rt-PA)
- Anistreplase
- Reteplase
- Tenecteplase.

Mechanism of Actions
- Activate tissue plasminogen activator (t-PA) → plasmin → lysis of blood clot
- Curative—Recanalization.

Uses
- Acute myocardial infarction (within 3 h, recanalization—50–90% cases)
- Deep vein thrombosis
- Pulmonary embolism
- Peripheral artery occlusion.

Antifibrinolytics
Drugs
- Epsilon-aminocaproic acid (EACA)
- Tranexamic acid.

Mechanism of Action
Combine with lysine binding sites of plasminogen and plasmin and prevent attachment of plasmin to the fibrin.

Uses
- Overdose of fibrinolytics
- Traumatic and surgical bleeding—Prostatic surgery, tooth extraction, tonsillectomy)
- Abruptio placenta, PPH, menorrhagia
- EACA—5 g oral/IV; tranexamic acid—1–1.5 g TDS oral.

Antiplatelet Drugs (Antithrombotic Drugs)
- Aspirin
- Dipyridamole

- Ticlopidine/clopidogrel
- Abciximab (GP IIb/IIIa antagonist).

Aspirin

Mechanism of Action

It inhibits COX and TX synthetase.

Dose

75–162 mg/day (commonly prescribed dose 81 mg/day).

Uses
- Myocardial infarction—Aspirin or aspirin + clopidogrel/dipyridamole
- Unstable angina—Aspirin/clopidogrel
- Coronary bypass implants—It is used to maintain patency of implanted vessels
- Prosthetic heart valves and hemodialysis patients
- Venous thromboembolism and peripheral vascular disease—As prophylaxis.
  Cerebrovascular transient ischemic attacks—Aspirin/clopidogrel.

Dipyridamole

Mechanism of Action

It inhibits phosphodiesterase and blocks uptake of adenosine to increase platelet cAMP → potentiate PGI_2 and inhibits platelet aggregation.

Ticlopidine/Clopidogrel

Mechanism of Action

It inhibits ADP and fibrinogen induced platelet aggregation.

Abciximab

Mechanism of Actions
- Glycoprotein (Gp) IIb/IIIa is adhesive receptor for fibrinogen and von Willebrand factor and helps in platelet aggregation.
- This receptor antagonist inhibits the above effect.

CHAPTER 3

Respiratory System

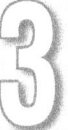

DRUGS USED IN BRONCHIAL ASTHMA, CHRONIC OBSTRUCTIVE PULMONARY DISEASE AND COUGH

Bronchial Asthma
- Asthma—Increased responsiveness of the tracheobronchial mucosa to various stimuli which results in widespread narrowing of the airways.
- Hallmarks—Cough, shortness of breath, chest tightness, wheezing.

Treatment

Classification of Drugs

- *Bronchodilators:*
    - Sympathomimetics:
        - Nonselective—Epinephrine, ephedrine
        - β_2-selective—Salbutamol (albuterol), terbutaline
        - New generation long-acting β_2-selective—Salmeterol and formoterol.
    - Methylxanthine—Theophylline, aminophylline.
    - Antimuscarinic agents—Ipratropium bromide (4-6 h), tiotropium (24 h).
- *Leukotrienes antagonists (LT D4-antagonists):* Zafirlukast and montelukast.
- *Mast cell stabilizers:* Cromolyn sodium (sodium cromoglycate), nedocromil
- *Corticosteroids:*
    - Systemic—Hydrocortisone, prednisolone
    - Inhalational—Beclomethasone, budesonide.
- *Anti-IgE monoclonal antibody (new approach):* Omalizumab.

Mechanism of Actions
- *Bronchodilators:*
  - Sympathomimetics
    - Adrenergic drugs cause bronchodilation through stimulation of β2-receptors → increase in cAMP → relaxation of bronchial muscles → bronchodilation
    - Fastest acting bronchodilators
  - Methylxanthines
    Mechanism of actions—
    - Inhibition of phosphodiesterase enzyme which is responsible for the degradation of cAMP or cGMP. So increase in cAMP → bronchodilation
    - Blockade of adenosine receptors → bronchodilation.
  - Antimuscarinic agents:
    - Ipratropium bromide(4–6 h), tiotropium (24 h)
    - Block the effect of acetylcholine on muscarinic receptors on bronchial smooth muscle → bronchodilation.
- *Leukotriene antagonists:* Zafirlukast and montelukast
  - Block the leukotriene D_4 receptors and prevent bronchoconstriction
    - Zileuton—5-lipoxygenase inhibitor → inhibits production of leukotrienes → bronchoconstriction is prevented.
- *Mast cell stabilizers:*
  - Cromolyn sodium (sodium cromoglycate)
  - Inhibits degranulation of mast cells → prevention of release of histamine → bronchoconstriction is prevented.
- *Corticosteroids:*
  - Reduce bronchial hyperactivity, mucosal edema, and suppresses the inflammation → bronchospasm is prevented
  - Spacer, gargling after each inhalation to decrease side effects.

Chronic Obstructive Pulmonary Disease (COPD)

- Progressive obstruction of airflow.
- Decline in airflow (FEV1)—Progressive and largely irreversible (unlike asthma)
- Causes—Cigarette smoking, environmental pollution, and occupational exposure (persons working in cement or cotton industries)
- COPD—Chronic bronchitis and emphysema

Management
Aims
- To lessen airflow obstruction
- To reduce respiratory symptoms and improve quality of life
- To prevent and treat secondary complications—Hypoxia, infections, and cor pulmonale.

Treatment Approaches
- Cessation of smoking (to prevent/slow the progression of disease)
- Acute exacerbation—Glucocorticoids provide some relief
- Among bronchodilators, muscarinic antagonists provide better result than $\rightarrow$ 2 agonists (due to high parasympathetic tone)
- Usually combination of ipratropium with short-acting $\rightarrow$ 2 agonist-better symptomatic relief.

Treatment
- Stop smoking
- Use of appropriate antimicrobial agent
- Bronchodilators—Salbutamol + ipratropium/oxitropium/tiotropium
- Oxygen therapy
- Theophylline—Adjunct to inhaled bronchodilators, positive inotropic (some value in cor pulmonale).

Cough
Cough is a protective reflex; occurs due to stimulation of mechano- or chemoreceptors; or stretch receptors.

Classifications
Coughs are of two types:
1. Nonproductive (useless)—Dry cough, no sputum, suppression is desirable
2. Productive (useful)—Expulsion of sputum, suppression is not desirable.

Treatment
- Specific therapy depends on etiology
- Nonspecific therapy/symptomatic therapy.

Specific Treatment Approach
Etiology
- Upper/lower respiratory tract infections
- Smoking/chronic bronchitis

- Pulmonary tuberculosis (TB)
- Asthmatic cough
- Gastroesophageal reflex.

Management
- Appropriate antibiotics
- Cessation of smoking/antibiotics
- Antitubercular drugs
- Bronchodilators/corticosteroids
- Omeprazole.

Symptomatic Therapy

Classifications
- Pharyngeal demulcents: It is used for dry cough
  - Lozenges, cough drops, linctuses.
- Expectorants (mucokinetics): It is used for productive cough
  - Sodium and potassium citrate
  - Potassium iodide
  - Bromhexine (mucolytics)
  - Guaifenesin
  - Dornase alfa (recombinant human deoxyribonuclease; used in cystic fibrosis; inhalational route)
  - N-acetyl cysteine.
- Antitussives (cough center suppressants): It is used for dry cough
  - Opioids: Codeine, pholcodine
  - Nonopioids: Noscapine, dextromethorphan
  - Antihistamines: Chlorpheniramine, diphenhydramine, promethazine.
- Pharyngeal demulcents:
  - They sooth throat and reduce afferent impulses from the inflamed/irritated pharyngeal mucosa and provide symptomatic relief in dry cough arising from throat.
  - Examples—Lozenges, linctuses, glycerin, cough drops.
- Expectorants (mucokinetics): These agents increase bronchial secretion and reduce its viscosity, facilitating its removal by coughing.

Mucolytics

Bromhexine—Obtained from adhatoda vasica
- Potent mucolytic and mucokinetic
- Induces thin copious bronchial secretion and increases mucociliary function (mucokinetic)

- Depolimerizes mucopolysaccharides directly as well as by liberating lysosomal enzymes—network of fibers in tenacious sputum is broken (mucolytic action).
  Adverse drug reactions
  - Rhinorrhea and lacrimation
  - Gastric irritation and hypersensitivity.
- *Antitussives (cough center suppressants):*
  - These drugs act in the CNS to raise the threshold of cough center or act peripherally in the respiratory tract to reduce cough impulses or have both actions.
  - It is used only for dry unproductive cough or if the cough is unduly tiring, disturbs sleep, or is hazardous (piles, hernia).
  Antihistamines
  - They relieve cough due to their sedative and anticholinergic actions, but lack selectivity for cough center.
  - They have no expectorant action.

Bronchodilators
- Bronchospasm can induce or aggravate cough.
- These agents relieve cough in patients with bronchoconstriction.
- Not routinely used.

ANTITUBERCULAR DRUGS
Tuberculosis
- Chronic granulomatous disease
- *Mycobacterium tuberculosis*
- *Mycobacterium avium*
- Multidrug-resistant TB (MDR-TB)

Antitubercular Drugs
First line: High efficacy, low toxicity, routinely used
Second line: Low efficacy, low toxicity, used occasionally.

First-line drugs	Second-line drugs	Newer drugs
Isoniazid	Thiacetazone	Cipro/oflo/moxifloxacin
Rifampin	Ethionamide	Azithro/clarithromycin
Pyrazinamide	Cycloserine	Rifabutin/rifapentine
Ethambutol	Kanamycin	Bedaquiline
	Amikacin	
	Streptomycin	

Alternative grouping of antitubercular drugs*		
Group I	First line oral anti-TB drugs	Isoniazid (INH), rifampin, pyrazinamide, ethambutol
Group II	Injectable anti-TB drugs	Streptomycin, kanamycin, amikacin, capreomycin
Group III	Fluoroquinolones	Ofloxacin, levofloxacin, mocifloxacin, ciprofloxacin
Group IV	Second line oral anti-TB drugs	Ethionamide, prothionamide, cycloserine, terizidone, para-aminosalicylic acid
Group V	Drugs with unclear efficacy*	Thiacetazone, clarithromycin, clofazimine, linezolid, amoxicillin/clavulanate, imipenem/cilastatin.

*Not recommended by WHO for routine use in MDR-TB patients.
Source: Adapted from Treatment of Tuberculosis Guidelines; WHO.

First-line Drugs
Isoniazid (Isonicotinic Acid Hydrazide, INH/H)

Mechanism of Actions
- It inhibits the synthesis of mycolic acids which are components of mycobacterial cell wall.
- Tuberculocidal.
- It acts on extracellular and intracellular tubercular bacilli; equally active in acidic and alkaline medium.

Adverse drug effects—
- It causes pyridoxine deficiency—Peripheral neuritis, paresthesia, numbness. So pyridoxine is given prophylactically to prevent neurological manifestations
- Hepatitis—High in older patients and alcoholics, rare in children.
- Rashes, fever, arthralgia

Rifampin (Rifampicin, R)
Mechanism of action—
Inhibits DNA-dependent RNA synthesis; tuberculocidal; acts on both extracellular and intracellular organisms.

Adverse drug reactions—
- Hepatitis
- Thrombocytopenia
- Respiratory syndrome—Breathlessness assessment with shock and collapse

- Purpura, hemolysis, renal failure
- Cutaneous syndrome—Flushing, pruritus, rash
- Flu-like syndrome—Chills, fever, headache
- Abdominal syndrome—Nausea, vomiting, abdominal cramps
- Urine—It may become orange-red—Harmless.

Other uses: Leprosy, prophylaxis of meningitis, brucellosis.

Pyrazinamide (Z)

Mechanism of action: Inhibits synthesis of mycolic acids; more active in acidic medium; highly lethal to intracellular organisms.

Adverse drug reaction: Hepatotoxicity, flushing, fever, arthralgia (hyperuricemia).

Contraindications—
- Patients with liver disease
- Patients with hyperuricemia—Gout can occur.

Ethambutol (E)

Mechanism of action: Probably inhibits arabinogalactan synthesis and interferes with mycolic acid incorporation in the cell wall; tuberculostatic.

Adverse drug reaction:
- Optic neuritis—Loss of visual acuity/color vision (contraindication— < 6 years in children)
  - Nausea, rashes, fever
  - Hyperuricemia.

Streptomycin(s)

Now it is considered as second line drug, however for academic convenience, it has been mentioned here.

Mechanism of action: Binds to 30S ribosome inside the bacteria and inhibits protein synthesis; tuberculocidal; acts only on extracellular bacilli.

Adverse drug reactions—
- Pain at injection site
- Ototoxicity, nephrotoxicity.

The offending drugs are given in decreasing order of frequency:
- Thrombocytopenia: R
- Neuropathy: H
- Vertigo: S

- Hepatitis: Z, R, H
- Rash: Z, R, E
- Neuropathy by isoniazid—Sensory neuropathy, H should be stopped; pyridoxine 50 mg tds; risk factors—diabetes, renal failure, alcoholism, malnutrition, pregnancy; pyridoxine 10 mg prophylactically.

Second-line Drugs

Thiacetazone
- Tuberculostatic; low efficacy
- Adverse drug reactions—Hepatitis and exfoliative dermatitis.

Para-aminosalicylic Acid (PAS)
- Similar to sulfonamide; tuberculostatic
- Adverse drug reactions—Anorexia, nausea, and epigastric pain.

Ethionamide
- Tuberculostatic
- Adverse drug reactions—Anorexia, nausea, and vomiting.

Cycloserine
- Chemical analog of D-alanine; inhibits cell wall synthesis; tuberculostatic
- Adverse drug reactions—CNS toxicity which leads to sleepiness, headache, tremor, and psychosis.

Kanamycin, Amikacin, Capreomycin
- More toxic antibiotics
- Reserved for rare cases not responding to usual therapy; or infection by atypical microbacteria.

Bedaquiline
- Mechanism: It inhibits mycobacterial ATP synthase (human ATP synthase is 20,000 times less sensitive)
- Metabolized by CYP3A4, t1/2- approx. 160 days
- Used in combination with other drugs in MDR-TB
- ADR: QT interval prolongation

Treatment Regimens
- Therapeutic goals:
  - To kill dividing bacilli
  - To kill persisting bacilli
  - To prevent emergence of resistance.

Respiratory System

- Drug combinations are selected to decrease the drug resistance together with consideration of cost convenience and feasibility.
- DOTS—Directly observed treatment short course—single daily dose of all the first line drugs is preferred—recommended by WHO in 1995.
- Short course chemotherapy (SCC).
- The conventional 12-18 months treatment has been replaced by more effective and less toxic 6-9 months duration.
- WHO (1997) has framed guidelines for different categories of TB patients.

All regimens have—
- Initial intensive phase—2-3 months; rapid killing of TB bacilli; symptomatic relief; sputum conversion.
- Continuation phase—4-6 months; remaining bacilli are eliminated so that relapse does not occur.

Categories of TB Patients and the Treatment Regimens (WHO, 2010) (Also Please Refer to the Government's Latest Guidelines of Your Country)

New Patient (Category I)
- New (untreated) smear positive pulmonary TB
- New smear negative pulmonary TB with extensive parenchymal involvement
- New cases of less severe/more severe forms of extra pulmonary TB, e.g., miliary TB, spinal TB, intestinal TB, etc.

Treatment Regimen
- Initial phase—2HRZE → HRZE daily for 2 months
- Continuation phase—4HR → HR daily for 4 months, so total duration 6 months.

Previously Treated Patients (Category II)
These are smear positive failure, relapse, and interrupted cases, become positive after completion of treatment.

Treatment Regimen
- Initial phase—2HRZES + 1HRZE → HRZES daily for 2 months followed by HRZE daily for 1 month
- Continuation phase—5 HRE → HRZE daily for 5 months, so total duration 8 months.

Multidrug-resistant TB
- It is defined as resistant to both H and R
- Extensively drug-resistant tuberculosis (XDR-TB)
- It is defined as MDR-TB that is resistant to quinolones and also to any one of kanamycin, capreomycin, or amikacin.

Treatment
- For H resistance
- RZE for 12 months
- For H + R resistance
- ZE + S/ethionamide + ciprofloxacin/ofloxacin.

TB in Pregnant Women
Six months regimen of 2HRZ + 4HR is given.

TB in Breastfeeding Women
- All anti-TB drugs are compatible with breastfeeding.
- Full course should be given to the mother.
- The infants should get BCG vaccination and isoniazid prophylaxis.

TB in AIDS Patients
Treatment regimen—2HRZE + 7HR.
- *Mycobacterium avium* complex (MAC)
- Clarithromycin + ethambutol ± rifabutin.
- Chemoprophylaxis

This is indicated only in:
- Contact of open cases showing recent Mantoux conversion
- Children with positive Mantoux and a TB patient in the family
- Neonate of tubercular mother.

Drugs
Combination of H (5 mg/kg) and R (10 mg/kg) given for 6 months.

Recommended Doses of First Line Antitubercular Drugs

Drugs	Doses	
	Daily (mg/kg)	3 × Per week (mg/kg)
Isoniazid (H)	5	10
Rifampin (R)	10	10
Pyrazinamide (Z)	25	35
Ethambutol (E)	15	30

HISTAMINE AND ANTIHISTAMINES

- Autacoids—Local hormones
    - Amine autacoids: Histamine, serotonin (5-hydroxytryptamine)
    - Lipid derived autacoids—PGs, LTs, PAF
    - Peptide autacoids: Plasmakinins (bradykinin, kallidin), angiotensin
- Histamine—Naturally occurring imidazole derivative
- Skin, GIT, mucosa, lungs, brain, CSF, bone marrow, body secretions, and venoms.
- Biosynthesis, storage, release, and metabolism
    - Histidine (decarboxylation)
    - In granules in mast cells (heparin and protein)
    - Exocytosis of granules (exchange with Na^+)
    - Degradation (oxidation and methylation)
- Histamine receptors
    - H1, H2, H3, and H4
    - G-protein coupled receptors
    - H3—Presynaptic (↓ release of histamine from histaminergic and other neurons)
    - H1 and H2—Postsynaptic (on cell membrane of neuroeffector junction)
    - H4—On blood cells (eosinophil, neutrophil, and CD4 T-cells)
    - H1 and H2 receptor agonists or antagonists—These are targets of drug research.

Characteristic Features of Histaminergic Receptors

Receptor	Location and function	Signal transduction	Agonists	Antagonists
H1	Smooth muscle-contraction (e.g. bronchoconstriction); BV vasodilation, ↑ Cap; Permeability; CNS-NT; sensory nerve endings pain, itching	GPCR→Gq →↑ IP_3/DAG	2-Methyl histamine	Mepyramine, triprolidine

Contd...

Contd...

Receptor	Location and function	Signal transduction	Agonists	Antagonists
H2	Gastric glands—acid secretion; BV—same as H1 function; heart—↑ HR, ↑FC Brain—NT	GPCR → Gs →↑ cAMP → phosphorylation of proteins	Dimaprit	Ranitidine, famotidine
H3	Brain presynaptic → ↓ histamine, NE, ACh release	GPCR → Gi → ↓ cAMP → ↓ Ca++ influx, K +channel opening	Imetit	Clobenpropit
H4	Eosinophil, neutrophil, CD4 T-cells-chemotaxis of WBC, production of blood cell types	GPCR → Gi → ↓cAMP → ↓ Ca+	Imetit, clozapine	Thioperamide

Pharmacological Actions of Histamine

- H1 receptor mediated actions
- Powerful stimulant of sensory nerve endings—Itching and pain (insects' bites and stings)
- Smooth muscles—Bronchoconstriction, spasmodic contractions of ileum and uterus, intestinal cramps, and diarrhea
- Exocrine glands (bronchioles, pancreas, salivary, and lacrimal) ↑ secretion
- Adrenal medulla— ↑ NE release (insignificant)
- Postsynaptic H1 in CNS—Maintenance of wakefulness.

H1 and H2 Receptor Mediated Actions

- Stimulation of H1 and H2 receptors → dilatation of arterioles and postcapillary venules → fall in BP, ↑ cap permeability, headache (stretching of sensory fibers around the cranial arteries); release of EDRF (NO)
- Heart—Positive chronotropic (H2); positive inotropic (H1 and H2)
- Response of intradermally injected histamine-triple response → immediate reddening of skin (flush→ dilatation of capillaries), formation of edematous patch (wheal → ↑ cap. permeability),

Respiratory System

and a red regular halo surrounding the wheal (flare → axon reflex causing vasodilatation).

Anaphylactic shock—Bronchospasm, angioneurotic edema, and hypotension.

H2 Receptor Mediated Actions
Powerful gastric acid secretion (H2 receptor on gastric parietal cells).

H1 Receptor Antagonists
First Generation
- Short to intermediate acting
- More sedating and are likely to have antimuscarinic side effects.

Second Generation
- Longer duration of action
- More selective H1 antagonism
- Poor permeability to BBB
- Additional antileukotriene and antiplatelet activating factor activity.

H1 Receptor Antagonists—First Generation

Name	Adult dose	Duration (h)	Anticho-linergic	Remarks
Highly sedative				
Dimenhydrinate	25–50 mg	4–6	+++	Antimotion sickness
Diphenhydramine	25–50 mg	4–6	+++	
Doxylamine	15–25 mg	4–6	++	Antiemetic
Hydroxyzine	25–50 mg	4–6	+++	Sleep aid
Promethazine	10–25 mg	4–6	+++	Antiemetic
Moderately				
Pheniramine	25–50 mg	4–6	+	
Cyproheptadine	4 mg	4–6	++	Antiserotonin
Cinnarizine	25–50 mg	4–6	++	
Meclizine	25–50 mg	12–20	++	
Buclizine	25–50 mg	4–6	++	
Mild				
Chlorpheniramine	4–8 mg	4–6	+	
Triprolidine	2.5–5 mg	4–6	+	Antimotion sickness
Cyclizine	25–50 mg	4–6	++	

Respiratory System

H1 Receptor Antagonists—Second Generation

Name	Adult dose	Duration (h)	Anti-cholinergic	Remarks
Astemizole	10 mg	24	–	
Fexofenadine	120-180 mg	12	–	
Cetirizine	10 mg	12–24	–	
Loratadine	10 mg	24	–	
Desloratadine	5 mg	24	–	Anti-inflammatory
Levocetirizine	5 mg	24		

Second generation drugs are nonsedating—Astemizole and terfenadine withdrawn in some countries because of cardiac toxicity (arrhythmias) when used with ketoconazole and erythromycin

Uses
- To prevent or treat allergic rhinitis
- As antiemetic (anticholinergic action)
    - Diphenhydramine, dimenhydrinate, cyclizine, meclizine (motion sickness)
    - Hydroxyzine, promethazine (antiemetic)
    - Doxylamine (morning sickness)
- Allergic conditions—Desloratadine
- In cough preparations.

Side Effects and Drug Interactions
- Sedation
- Antimuscarinic effects: Dry mouth, urinary retention, constipation.

Drug Interactions
- With alcohol and other CNS depressants → more sedation (impaired alertness and psychomotor skill)
- With antimuscarinic drugs and tricyclic antidepressants → more antimuscarinic side effects
- Astemizole and terfenadine with ketoconazole, chloramphenicol, and erythromycin (enzyme inhibitors) → cardiac arrhythmias (torsades de pointes).

Fexofenadine (active metabolite of terfenadine) does not produce torsades de pointes.

NASAL DECONGESTANTS
Drugs that Relieve Nasal Congestion
Work by reducing swelling of the mucous membranes in the nasal passages.
- Nasal decongestants should only be used by patients for a maximum of 3 days, because rebound congestion may occur in the form of rhinitis medicamentosa.
- These drugs are a common form of nasal relief, due to their quick effects which can clear the sinus in as little as 10 seconds.

Mechanism of Action
Topical decongestants are vasoconstrictors, and work by constricting the blood vessels within the nasal cavity.

Nasal decongestants are:
- Ephedrine
- Oxymetazoline
- Phenylephrine
- Pseudoephedrine
- Tramazoline
- Xylometazoline
- Naphazoline.

Adverse Drug Reactions
- Hypertension
- Sleeplessness
- Anxiety
- Dizziness
- Excitability
- Nervousness.
- Decongestants are normally paired with antihistamines to lessen this effect, but the combination of both classes of drugs does not necessarily cancel the side effects of each other.
- Topical nasal or ophthalmic decongestants quickly develop tachyphylaxis (a rapid decrease in the response to a drug after repeated doses over a short period of time). Long-term use is not recommended since these agents lose effectiveness after a few days.

CHAPTER 4

Musculoskeletal System

NONSTEROIDAL ANTI-INFLAMMATORY DRUGS (NSAIDs)

- Analgesics are of two types:
  1. Narcotic
  2. Nonsteroidal
- Anti-inflammatory drugs are of two types:
  1. Steroidal—Corticosteroids
  2. Nonsteroidal
- Nonsteroidal analgesics are more effective in pain associated with inflammation/musculoskeletal origin.

Classification of NSAIDs

- Nonselective cyclooxygenase (COX) inhibitors
  - Salicylates—Aspirin, diflunisal
  - Pyrazolone derivatives—Phenylbutazone and oxyphenbutazone
  - Propionic acid derivatives—Ibuprofen, naproxen, ketoprofen, flurbiprofen
  - Anthranilic acid derivatives—Mefenamic acid
    - Arylacetic acid derivative—Diclofenac
    - Oxicam derivatives—Piroxicam, tenoxicam
    - Pyrrolopyrrole derivative—Ketorolac
- Selective COX-2 inhibitors—Celecoxib, rofecoxib, valdecoxib, and etoricoxib.
- Analgesic, antipyretic with poor anti-inflammatory effect
  - Para-aminophenol derivative—Paracetamol
  - Pyrazolone derivatives—Metamizole
  - Benzoxazocine derivative—Nefopam
- NSAID which does not inhibit prostaglandin (PG) synthesis—Nefopam.

Musculoskeletal System

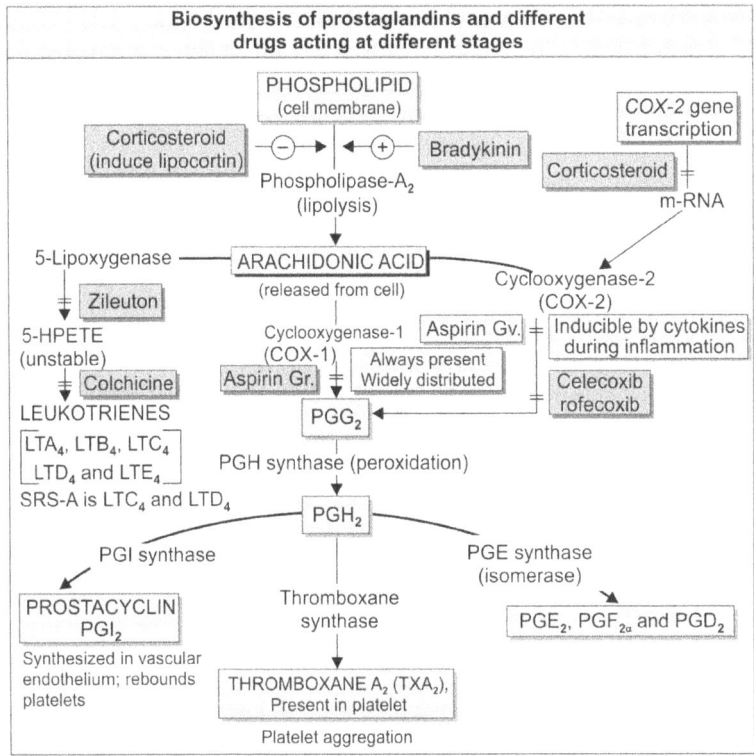

Biosynthesis of prostaglandins and different drugs acting at different stages

Actions/Features of NSAIDs
- Analgesic
- Antipyretic
- Anti-inflammatory
- Antiplatelet aggregatory
- Gastric mucosal damage
- Renal salt/water retention
- Delay/prolongation of labor
- Ductus arteriosus closure
- Aspirin sensitive asthma precipitation.

Beneficial Effects due to Prostaglandin Synthesis Inhibition
- Analgesic—Prevention of pain nerve ending sensitization
- Antipyresis
- Anti-inflammatory
- Antithrombotic (aspirin)
- Closure of ductus arteriosus.

Toxicities due to Prostaglandin Synthesis Inhibition
- Gastric mucosal damage—Peptic ulcer, bleeding
- Bleeding—Inhibition of platelet function
- Limitation of renal blood flow—Na^+ and water retention
- Delay/prolongation of labor
- Asthma and anaphylactoid reactions in susceptible individuals.

Adverse Effects of NSAIDs
- Gastrointestinal—Peptic ulceration, gastric bleeding
- Renal—Na^+ and water retention, analgesic nephropathy (renal papillary necrosis), renal failure
- Hematological—Bleeding, thrombocytopenia
- Others—Asthma exacerbation, skin rashes, pruritus, and mental confusion.

Precautions and Contraindications
- Peptic ulcer
- In children suffering from viral infection (aspirin is contraindicated due to fear of Reye's syndrome, so do not use aspirin in viral fevers as antipyretic agent)
- Chronic liver disease
- Congestive heart failure (CHF)
- Pregnancy (low birth weight babies, delayed/prolonged labor, greater PPH, premature closure of ductus arteriosus)
- Aspirin may have to be stopped 1 week before surgery to minimize a risk of bleeding.

Uses
- As analgesic—Headache, backache, myalgia, joint pain, pulled muscle, toothache, and dysmenorrhea (aspirin: 0.3-0.6 g 6-8 hourly).
- As antipyretic—Paracetamol is preferred
- Acute rheumatic fever—Aspirin 3-6 g/day
- Rheumatoid arthritis (RA)—Aspirin 3-5 g/day
- Osteoarthritis
- Postmyocardial infarction and poststroke patients—Aspirin 75-162 mg/day (commonly 81 mg/day)
- Preeclampsia—Aspirin
- Acute gout—Naproxen, indomethacin, diclofenac
- Closure of patent ductus arteriosus—Indomethacin, aspirin
- Ankylosing spondylitis.

DRUGS USED IN THE TREATMENT OF RHEUMATOID ARTHRITIS AND GOUT

Treatment of Rheumatoid Arthritis

Classification of Drugs

- Disease-modifying antirheumatic drugs (DMARDs):
  - Methotrexate
  - Hydroxychloroquine and chloroquine
  - Leflunomide
  - Minocycline
  - Sulfasalazine
  - Cyclosporine
  - Gold compounds (oral—auranofin)
  - D-penicillamine (chelating compound)
- Corticosteroids
- Newer drugs (biologic response modifiers):
  - Anti-TNFα—Etanercept, infliximab, adalimumab, certolizumab pegol, and golimumab
  - Binds to CD80/86 antigen—Abatacept
  - Antibody against CD20 antigen—Rituximab
  - Antibody against IL6 receptor—Tocilizumab
  - Oral inhibitor of Janus Kinase—Tofacitinib
  - IL1 receptor antagonist—Anakinra
- NSAIDs, e.g., aspirin.

Disease-modifying Antirheumatic Drugs

Gold

- ↓ Chemotaxis, phagocytosis, macrophage and lysosomal activity, and cell-mediated immunity (CMI)
- It is used with NSAIDs
- Auranofin (orally active gold compound—29% gold)
- Adverse drug reactions—Diarrhea and abdominal cramps.

Chloroquine/Hydroxychloroquine

- Exact mechanism of action—Not known
- However, ↓ Interleukin-1 (IL-1)
- Adverse drug reactions—Retinal damage and corneal opacity, and cardiac toxicity (arrhythmias).

Sulfasalazine

- Sulfonamide group of antibiotic
- It is split into 5-aminosalicylic acid (5-ASA) + sulfapyridine by colonic bacteria

- 5-aminosalicylic acid (5-ASA)—Ulcerative colitis
- Sulfapyridine—Rheumatoid arthritis
- ↓ Cytokine production and superoxide radicals → ↓ inflammation.

Immunosuppressants

Methotrexate
- Potent immunosuppressant and anti-inflammatory property
- ↓ Cytokine production, chemotaxis, and CMI.

Azathioprine
↓ Differentiation and function of T-cells, and natural killer cells → ↓ CMI.

Cyclosporine
- T-cell specific → ↓ CMI
- High renal toxicity → reserved for refractory cases.

Corticosteroids (Adjuvant)
- These have potent immunosuppressant and anti-inflammatory properties (due to ↓ production of cytokine, ↓ function of leukocytes).
- These are used with NSAIDs ± DMARD.
- For example, prednisolone, cortisone, hydrocortisone.

Newer Drugs (Biologic Response Modifiers)

IL-1, IL-6, and TNFα are involved in the inflammatory response (cell stimulation, proliferation, maturation, chemotaxis, and destruction). Inhibition of these cytokines leads to decreased inflammation and inhibition of the disease progression. Janus kinase is the receptor for the different cytokines, so inhibition of this receptor leads to blockade of cytokine functions. CD20 is involved in immune cell activation; blockade leads to decreased activation of immune cells. CD80/86 (antigen presenting cell) binds with CD28 of T-cell and is required for costimulation (signal 2) of helper T-cells.

DMARDs have been shown to slow the course of the disease, induce remission, and prevent further destruction of the joints and involved tissues. When a patient is diagnosed with RA, DMARDs should be started immediately to help stop the progression of the disease at the earlier stages. Usually methotrexate with etanercept or with any other biologic response modifier in combination is used.

Treatment of Gout

- Acute gout
  NSAIDs—Indomethacin, naproxen, and piroxicam
  Colchicine
  Corticosteroids.
- Chronic gout
  Uricosurics
  - Probenecid, sulfinpyrazone.
  Synthesis inhibitor
  - Allopurinol, febuxostat
  Recombinant urate-oxidase or uricase (uricase converts uric acid into allantoin which is water soluble and easily excreted)
  - Pegloticase (in chronic gout), rasburicase (in tumor lysis syndrome).

Acute Gout

Colchicine

- Mechanism of action:
  - ↓ Release of glycoprotein from inflammatory cells → ↓ lactic acid production; ↓ release of lysosomal enzymes
  - Binds to tubulin (fibrillar protein) and inhibits granulocyte migration to the inflamed joint.
- Other actions: Antimitotic and ↑ gut motility.
- Adverse reactions

At Lower Dose
Vomiting and diarrhea (very common, may occur in 50% patients).

At Higher Dose
- Kidney damage, CNS depression
- Muscular paralysis and respiratory failure.

Corticosteroids
- Intra-articular injection
- Systemic steroids.

Chronic Gout

Uricosuric Drugs
- Block tubular reabsorption of uric acid → ↑ uric acid level
- For example, probenecid, sulfinpyrazone

- Probenecid also ↓ excretion of penicillins, cephalosporins and nitrofurantoin
- Salicylates block uricosuric action of probenecid.

Uric Acid Synthesis Inhibitor
- Allopurinol:
  - Inhibits xanthine oxidase, an enzyme necessary for uric acid synthesis.
  - Metabolite of allopurinol → alloxanthine is longer acting and inhibits xanthine oxidase noncompetitively.
- Febuxostat:
  - It also inhibits xanthine oxidase; more potent and effective than allopurinol.

SKELETAL MUSCLE RELAXANTS

Drugs which act on skeletal muscle fall into two major therapeutic groups.

Neuromuscular Blocking Agents
- These are used during surgical procedures and intensive care units to cause paralysis.
- These interfere with transmission at the neuromuscular junction and primarily used as adjunct to general anesthesia.

Spasmolytics
They are used to reduce the spasticity in a variety of neurologic conditions, also called centrally acting muscle relaxants, e.g., diazepam, baclofen.
- Neuromuscular blocking drugs:
  - Nondepolarizing/antagonist type/competitive blockers
    - Long-acting (30–120 min)—d-tubocurarine, pancuronium, doxacurium, pipecuronium
    - Intermediate-acting (30–60 min)—Vecuronium, atracurium, cisatracurium, rocuronium
    - Short-acting (10–20 min)—Mivacurium, rapacurium.
  - Depolarizing/agonist type blockers (3–6 min)
    - Succinylcholine (suxamethonium), decamethonium
- Directly acting muscle relaxant: Dantrolene sodium.
- Centrally acting muscle relaxants/spasmolytic drugs: Diazepam, baclofen, tizanidine, chlorzoxazone.

Neuromuscular Blocking Drugs

Nondepolarizing Drugs

Curare—Initially used by South American as arrow poison to kill the animals, the active component was d-tubocurarine, and it was first used clinically in 1930.

Mechanism of Actions

- Cause competitive block, can be reversed by acetylcholinesterase inhibitors.
- Tubocurarine is considered as the prototype of this neuromuscular blocking group.
- This group of drugs act at the nicotinic receptor site (Nm) by competing with acetylcholine.

Depolarizing Drugs

Mechanism of Actions

Phase I block (depolarizing phase)—

- They bind to the nicotinic receptors (Nm) and depolarize muscle end-plates by opening the sodium channels. Muscle fasciculations may occur.

Phase II block (desensitizing phase)—

- It is slow in onset and results from desensitization of Nm cholinoceptors though the membrane becomes repolarized.
- Nearly identical to the nondepolarizing blockade, can partly be reversed by acetylcholinesterase inhibitors.

Pharmacokinetics

All neuromuscular blockers are quaternary ammonium compounds-polarized, so not absorbed orally, given through IV or IM.

They do not cross placenta or penetrate brain. They are metabolized in liver and some of them are metabolized by plasma cholinesterase/pseudocholinesterase/butyrylcholinesterase, e.g. mivacurium, succinylcholine.

Spontaneous breakdown (Hofmann elimination)—Atracurium.

Scoline Apnea

- Due to genetically variant plasma cholinesterase; decreased affinity to succinylcholine and fails to metabolize; prevalence 1:3000.
- Continuous apnea for 2-3 hours; no treatment is available; mechanical ventilation should be provided till the recovery occurs.

Actions

Skeletal Muscle—Flaccid Paralysis
- Histamine release—d-tubocurarine, atracurium, mivacurium
- Hypotension, flushing, bronchospasm, increased respiratory secretions.

Cardiovascular Effects
- Competitive blockers-Due to ganglionic blockade, histamine release, reduced venous return (result of paralysis)
  - Hypotension and tachycardia.
- Succinylcholine—Cardiac arrhythmias may occur when administered with halothane anesthetic agent.
- GIT—It may enhance postoperative paralytic ileus.
- Central nervous system (CNS)—Do not cross blood-brain barrier (BBB), no central effects.

Other Adverse Effects of Depolarizing Blockade
- Hyperkalemia (burns, head injury, trauma—These conditions are also associated with increased potassium level). So, succinylcholine is contraindicated in these situations, and rocuronium is used. Succinylcholine— ↑ blood K^+ during first phase of depolarization. Cardiac arrest may occur.
- Increased intraocular pressure (contraction of myofibrils or transient dilation of choroidal vessels)—Declines after 5 minutes.
- Increased intragastric pressure (due to fasciculations), emesis more likely.
- Muscle pain (secondary to the unsynchronized contractions of adjacent muscle fibers just before the onset of paralysis).

Interaction with Other Drugs
- Anesthetics—Inhaled anesthetics augment the neuromuscular blockade.
- Antibiotics—Aminoglycosides enhance the blockade.
- Local anesthetic and antiarrhythmic drugs enhance the neuromuscular block.

Uses
- *Surgical relaxation as an adjunct to general anesthesia:* Intra-abdominal and intrathoracic surgery—Succinylcholine is employed for brief procedure—Endotracheal intubation, laryngoscopy, bronchoscopy, esophagoscopy, reduction of fractures and dislocations, electroconvulsive therapy.

- *Control of ventilation:* In ICU patients who have ventilatory failure, neuromuscular blocking drugs are given to facilitate mechanical ventilation.
- *Treatment of convulsions:* Severe cases of tetanus, status epilepticus (not controlled by diazepam), convulsions in local anesthetic toxicity.

Centrally Acting Muscle Relaxants
Mechanism of action—Inhibit spinal and supraspinal polysynaptic reflexes involved in regulation of muscle tone.

Uses
- Acute muscle spasms (e.g., sprain, dislocations)
- Torticollis
- Spastic neurological disease—Hemiplegia, paraplegia, multiple sclerosis, cerebral palsy
- Tetanus
- Electroconvulsive therapy.

Directly Acting Muscle Relaxant
- Dantrolene sodium—Inhibits Ca^{++} release from sarcoplasmic reticulum
- Use—Malignant hyperthermia
- Adverse drug reactions—Muscle weakness, diarrhea, and liver toxicity.

Cardiovascular System

CHAPTER 5

HYPERTENSION

Treatment of Hypertension
- BP = Cardiac output (CO) × Total peripheral resistance (TPR)
- Address sympathetic overactivity
- Address overactive renin-angiotensin-aldosterone system.

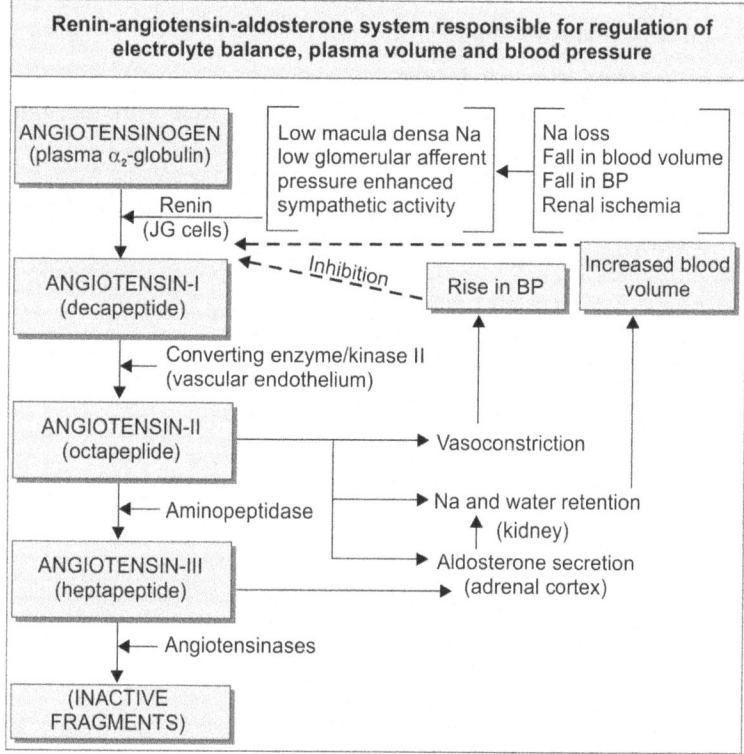

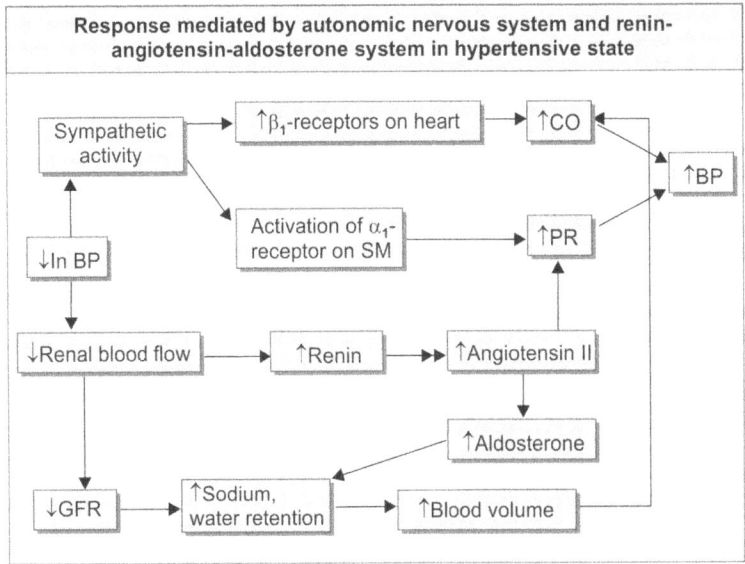

Classification of Hypertension

Category	SBP (mm Hg)	DBP
Normal	<120	<80
Prehypertension	120–139	80–89
Hypertension	≥ 140	≥ 90
• Stage 1	140–159	90–99
• Stage 2	≥ 160	≥ 100

(SBP: systolic blood pressure; DBP: diastolic blood pressure)

Classification of Drugs

- Angiotensin converting enzyme
  - Captopril, enalapril
- Angiotensin antagonists
  - Losartan, valsartan
- Calcium channel blockers
  - Verapamil, diltiazem, nifedipine, amlodipine
- Diuretics
  - Thiazide—Hydrochlorothiazide
  - High ceiling—Furosemide
  - K^+ sparing—Spironolactone

- β-adrenergic blockers: Propranolol, atenolol (beta-1 selective blockers are preferred)
- β + α-adrenergic blockers: Labetalol, carvedilol
- α-adrenergic blockers: Prazosin, phentolamine
- Centrally acting: Clonidine, methyldopa
- Vasodilators: Hydralazine, minoxidil, sodium nitroprusside

ACE Inhibitors
Mechanism of Action
These agents inhibit the conversion of angiotensin I to angiotensin II—Fall in BP.

Adverse Drug Reactions
- Dry cough
- Angioedema
- Hypotension
- Hyperkalemia.

Contraindication
Pregnancy: Renal artery stenosis (bilateral or unilateral solitary).

Angiotensin Antagonists
Mechanism of Action
Block the angiotensin II receptors.

Adverse Drug Reactions
- Hypotension
- Hyperkalemia
- Headache, dizziness.

Contraindication
Pregnancy.

Calcium Channel Blockers
Mechanism of Action
- They block Ca^{++} channels; most important actions are:
  - Smooth muscle relaxation
  - Negative chronotropic, inotropic, and dromotropic action on heart.

Adverse Drug Reactions
- Nausea, constipation, bradycardia
- Hypotension

Diuretics

Mechanism of Action

Diuretics →↓ water and sodium retention →↓ blood volume →↓ CO ↓ BP

- *Side effects:*
  - Hyperuricemia
  - Hypokalemia (except K^+ sparing diuretics)
  - Hyperglycemia
  - Hyperlipidemia.
- *Other uses:*
  - Edema
  - Pulmonary edema
  - Cerebral edema
  - Forced diuresis.

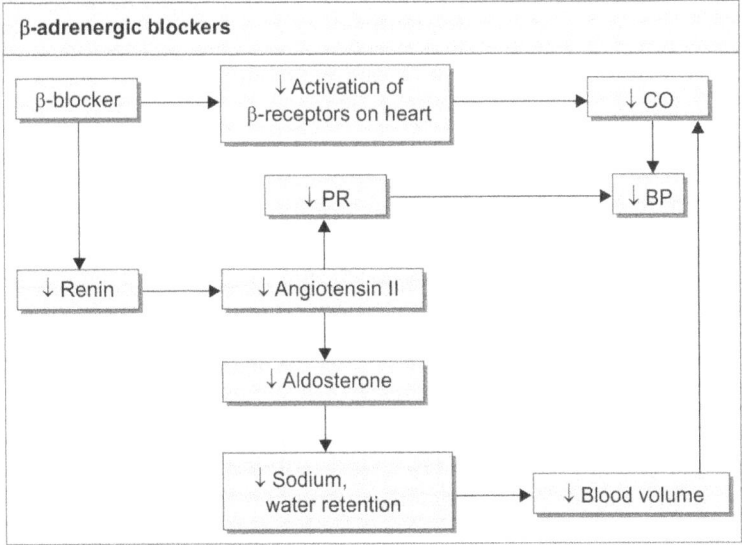

(PR: peripheral resistance; CO: cardiac output; BP: blood pressure)

Adverse Drug Reactions

- CNS effects—Fatigue, lethargy, insomnia
- Hallucinations
- ↓ Libido and impotence—Sexual dysfunction
- Disturb lipid metabolism
- Rebound hypertension (if discontinued suddenly).

Centrally Acting (Central Sympatholytics)
Clonidine (α_2-agonist) → decrease sympathetic outflow→ fall in BP.

Adverse Drug Reactions
- Insomnia, depression
- Impotence
- Bradycardia
- Postural hypotension
- Rebound hypertension
- Sedation, dry mouth.

Vasodilators
Mechanism of Action
Release of endothelium dependent relaxing factor (EDRF later known as nitric oxide—NO)→ relaxation of vascular smooth muscle cells → vasodilatation → fall in BP.

Adverse Drug Reactions
- Headache
- Palpitation
- Angina
- Edema, nasal stuffiness.

Treatments
- First-line drugs—ACE inhibitors/angiotensin II type 1 receptor antagonists, CCBs, diuretics
- Start with a single drug.

Stage Two—Combination of Drugs
- Diuretics/vasodilators/CCBs/ACE inhibitors + β-blockers
- Sympathetic inhibitors/vasodilators + diuretic
- ACE inhibitors/AT1 antagonists + diuretics
- ACE inhibitors + CCB or β-blocker
- β-blocker + prazosin.

ANTIANGINAL DRUGS

Drugs that prevent or terminate attack of angina pectoris.

Angina Pectoris
Sudden and severe substernal pain due to an imbalance between myocardial oxygen demand and supply by coronary vessels.

Types of Angina Pectoris
- Stable/classical/atherosclerotic angina
  - Underlying pathology—Atherosclerosis
  - Precipitated by—Exercise, emotion, stress, cold, coitus.
- Variant/Prinzmetal's angina
  - Underlying pathology—Transient vasospasm of coronary blood vessels + atheroma
  - Unpredictable; during rest or sleep.
- Unstable/crescendo angina: Ruptured atherosclerotic plaque.

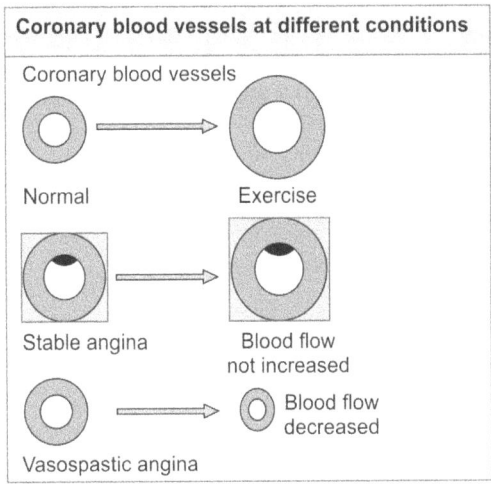

Classification of Drugs
- Nitrates
  - Short acting—Glyceryl trinitrate (GTN, nitroglycerin)
  - Long acting—Isosorbide dinitrate, isosorbide mononitrate, erythrityl tetranitrate, pentaerythritol tetranitrate.
- β-blockers—Propranolol, metoprolol, atenolol
- Ca^{++} channel blockers
  - Phenylalkylamine—Verapamil
  - Benzothiazepine—Diltiazem
  - Dihydropyridine—Nifedipine, felodipine, amlodipine, nimodipine.

Clinical Classifications
- To terminate attack—GTN, isosorbide dinitrate (sublingually).
- For prophylaxis—All other drugs; low dose aspirin.

Nitrates

Mechanism of Action
Nitrates → nitric oxide (inside smooth muscle cell) → activates cytosolic guanylyl cyclase → ↑ cGMP → dephosphorylation of myosin light chain kinase (MLCK) → ↓ activation of myosin → smooth muscle relaxation → vasodilatation.

Adverse Drug Reactions
- Throbbing headache; fullness in head (due to dilatation of meningeal vessels).
- Flushing, sweating, weakness, palpitation, dizziness, fainting.
- Postural hypotension.
- Methemoglobinemia → ↓ oxygen carrying capacity; anemia → caution).
- Rashes—Rare
  - Contraindication—In increased ICP.

Tolerance
- Continuous use → ineffective or ↓ in response
- At least 8 h/day—Free of drug.

Dependence
- Sudden withdrawal after prolonged use → spasm of coronary and peripheral blood vessels.
- Withdrawal should be gradual.

Interaction
Nitrates + other vasodilators → severe hypotension, myocardial infarction (MI), and death.

Glyceryl Trinitrate
- Volatile liquid → absorbed in inert matrix → tablet → tight glass container.
- Sublingual route → effects within 1-2 minutes; to terminate anginal attack.
- Intravenous (IV) route—Unstable angina, coronary vasospasm, LVF with MI, HTN, during cardiac surgery.

Uses
- Angina pectoris
- CHF and acute LVF
- MI
- Cardiac procedure (e.g., percutaneous coronary angioplasty)

- Biliary colic
- Esophageal spasm
- Cyanide poisoning: Hb + sodium nitrite (weak vasodilator)

10 mL of 3% solution → methemoglobin + cyanide → cyanomethemoglobin + sodium thiosulfate (50 ml of 25% solution) → methemoglobin + sodium thiocyanate → excreted in urine. Second approach to treat cyanide poisoning: Hydroxocobalamin (vit B12); hydroxocobalamin + cyanide → cyanocobalamin → excreted in urine.

TREATMENT OF CONGESTIVE CARDIAC FAILURE (CCF)

Congestive Cardiac Failure
- Inability of the heart to generate cardiac output sufficient for the body's needs
- Insufficient oxygenated blood
- Increased venous pressure—Edema
- Decreased excitation—Contraction coupling process.

Types
- Forward failure
- Backward failure
- Systolic dysfunction
- Diastolic dysfunction
- Right-sided failure
- Left-sided failure
- Low-output failure
- High-output failure.

Primary Signs and Symptoms
- Tachycardia
- Decreased exercise tolerance and fatigue
- Shortness of breath
- Peripheral and pulmonary edema
- Cardiomegaly.

Causes
- Ischemic heart disease
- Hypertension
- Valvular heart disease
- Dilated cardiomyopathy
- Congenital heart disease.

Cardiovascular System

Pathophysiology of Heart Failure
Compensatory reflexes:
- Activation of neurohormonal (extrinsic) mechanism
  - Sympathetic activation
  - Renin-angiotensin-aldosterone system activation.
- Cardiac compensation (intrinsic)
  - Increase in volume and pressure
  - Remodeling
  - Myocardial hypertrophy.

Pathophysiology of Cardiac Performance
- ↑ Preload—Salt restriction, diuretics, and venodilators.
- ↑ Afterload—Arteriolar dilators.
- ↓ Contractility—Inotropic drugs.

Drugs
- Inotropes
  - Cardiac glycosides—Digoxin and digitoxin
  - β-agonists—Dobutamine, dopamine
  - PDE-III—Inamrinone and milrinone.
- Diuretics
  - Loop diuretics, thiazides, K$^+$ sparing diuretics.
- Vasodilators
  - Arteriolar—Hydralazine, Ca^{++} channel blockers
  - Venous—Nitrates
  - Both—ACE inhibitors, angiotensin receptor blockers.
- β-blockers
  - Bisoprolol, carvedilol (additional α1), metoprolol.

Cardiac glycosides—Digoxin and Digitoxin

(*Note:* Digitoxin is no longer used because of its unfavorable pharmacokinetic properties)

Mechanism of action—It inhibits Na$^+$-K$^+$ ATPase →↑ intracellular Na$^+$ →↑ intracellular Ca^{++} →↑ interaction of actin and myosin →↑ contractility.

Adverse Drug Reactions
- GIT—Nausea, vomiting, and diarrhea
- CNS—Disorientation, hallucination, stimulation of CTZ
- Eye—Visual disturbances (color perception → yellowish vision).

Management of Heart Failure
- Acute heart failure
  - Diuretics
  - Vasodilators
  - Inotropes.
- Chronic heart failure.

Steps
- Reduce workload of heart
  - Limit activity level
  - Reduce weight
  - Control hypertension
- Restrict salt
- Give ACE inhibitors
- Give diuretics (spironolactone)
- Give digitalis if systolic dysfunction or atrial fibrillation
- Give β-blockers in stable patients.

DRUGS USED IN RHEUMATIC FEVER AND MYOCARDIAL INFARCTION
Rheumatic Fever
- Inflammatory disease—After an infection with *Streptococcus* bacteria (sore throat or scarlet fever)
- Organs involved—Heart, joints, skin, brain
- Cross reaction to human connective tissue.

Clinical Features
Fever, anorexia, cardiac problems (dyspnea, chest pain), joint pain, arthritis (knees, elbows, ankles, wrists), skin nodules, skin rash (erythema marginatum), Sydenham chorea (quick and uncoordinated jerky movements).

Diagnosis—Jones Criteria
- Major—Carditis, polyarthritis, chorea, erythema marginatum, subcutaneous nodules
- Minor—Fever, arthralgia, ↑ erythrocyte sedimentation rate (ESR) or C-reactive proteins (CRP), leukocytosis, first or second degree heart block.

Two Major or One Major + Two Minor Criteria → Rheumatic Fever
- Chronic rheumatic heart disease (RHD)
- 50% of patients who develop carditis → mitral valve stenosis (>90%) (because of fibrosis).

Cardiovascular System

Management
- Bed rest (because of dyspnea and carditis).
- Aspirin—Arthritis → decreases within 24 h; 60-120 mg/kg not exceeding 8 g/day.
- Corticosteroids—Rapid symptomatic relief; prescribed in severe cases of carditis and arthritis; prednisolone or prednisone 1-2 mg/kg/day.

Subsequent Prophylaxis
- Benzathine penicillin 1.2 MU IM every 4 weeks till 18 years of age or 5 years after an attack, whichever is more.

OR
- Phenoxymethyl penicillin 500 mg → 5 years after the last attack until patient reaches 20 years of age
- If allergic to penicillin → erythromycin.

Myocardial Infarction
- Ischemic necrosis of a portion of myocardium
- Occlusion of branch of coronary artery
- 25% of patients die before therapy.

Clinical Features
- Chest pain → tightness, pressure, squeezing
- Pain—It may radiate → jaw, neck, arms (left →↑), back and epigastrium
- Nausea, cough
- Anxiety, lightheadedness
- Diaphoresis
- Palpitation
- Loss of consciousness and sudden death.

Diagnosis
- History
- Physical examination
- Tests—ECG, chest X-ray, blood tests—Cardiac markers → creatinine kinase—MB, troponin I and T; coronary angiography.

Risk Factors
- Diabetes
- Smoking
- Hypercholesterolemia
- Hypertension

- Family history of ischemic heart disease
- Obesity (BMI > 30 kg/m^2)
- Age—Male > 45 years; Female > 55 years
- Stress
- Sedentary lifestyle
- Heavy alcoholism.

Management
- To relieve pain, anxiety, and apprehension—Opioid analgesic (morphine, pethidine), diazepam.
- Maintenance of oxygenation—O_2 inhalation.
- Maintenance of blood volume and tissue perfusion—Slow IV infusion of normal saline (avoid volume overload).
- Correction of acidosis (due to lactic acid)—IV infusion of sodium bicarbonate.
- Prevention and treatment of arrhythmia—β-blocker.
- Pump failure (ventricular failure)
  - Furosemide
  - Vasodilators—Arteriolar, venous, or combined
  - Inotropic drugs—Dobutamine, dopamine.
- Thrombolytics (to dissolve the clot)—Streptokinase/urokinase/alteplase.
- Prevention of thrombus extension—Heparin followed by oral anticoagulant.
- Prevention of cardiac remodeling and subsequent coronary heart disease—ACE inhibitors.
- Prevention of future attacks (prophylaxis)
  - Low dose aspirin (75–162 mg/day) →↓ platelet aggregation
  - β-blocker—Atenolol (↓ reinfarction)
    Hypolipidemic drugs—Lovastatin, simvastatin, fenofibrate (→↓ hyperlipidemia)
  - Regular exercise (at least 10–15 minutes brisk walk/day).

ANTIARRHYTHMIC DRUGS

Classifications
- Class I (membrane stabilizing agents)
  - A—Quinidine, procainamide
  - B—Lignocaine
  - C—Propafenone
- Class II (β-blockers)—Propranolol, sotalol, esmolol

- Class III (widening AP)—Amiodarone
- Class IV (Ca^{++} channel blockers)—Verapamil, diltiazem.

In addition:
- For paroxysmal supraventricular tachycardia (PSVT)—Adenosine
- For atrioventricular (AV) block—Isoprenaline, atropine
- AF, AFl, PSVT—Digitalis (to control ventricular rate).

Class I Drugs
- These drugs limit the conduction of sodium channels across cell membrane → local anesthetic agent.
- They interfere with depolarization and decrease responsive to excitation.

Subclass IA
Quinidine, procainamide, disopyramide.

Mechanism of Actions
- Block activated Na^+ channels
- Quinidine has additional class III properties.

Quinidine
Adverse Drug Reactions
- Gastrointestinal intolerance
- Cinchonism—Ringing in ears, deafness, vertigo, visual disturbances
- Idiosyncrasy and hypersensitivity reactions.

Interaction
- Quinidine + digoxin— ↑ digoxin toxicity
- Quinidine + diuretics—Hypokalemia
- Quinidine + vasodilators—↓ BP → syncope
- Quinidine + verapamil/β-blockers—cardiac depression.

Subclass IB
Lignocaine, mexiletine.

Mechanism of Action
Block Na^+ channels in inactivated states.

Adverse Drug Reactions of Lignocaine (Lidocaine)
- Mainly the dose-related neurological effects—Drowsiness, nausea, paresthesia, blurred vision, twitching and fits
- Cardiac depression and hypotension (at higher dose).

Cardiovascular System

Uses
- Ventricular tachycardia
- Local anesthetic agent.

Subclass IC
Propafenone, flecainide.

Mechanism of Actions
- Most potent Na⁺ channels blockers (mainly in open state)
- Delay conduction in the bypass tract of Wolff-Parkinson-White (WPW) syndrome
- Reserve drug for ventricular arrhythmias.

Adverse Drug Reactions
- Sudden cardiac death
- Gastrointestinal disturbances
- Visual disturbances.

Class II
Propranolol, sotalol, esmolol.

Mechanism of Actions
- Suppress adverse drug reactions energetically mediated ectopic activity
- Highly effective in arrhythmias seen in pheochromocytoma and during anesthesia with halothane.

Class III
Amiodarone.

Mechanism of Action
↑ repolarization and ERP, tissue remains refractory even after full repolarization.

Uses
Resistant ventricular tachycardia (VT) and recurrent ventricular fibrillation (VF).

Adverse Drug Reactions
- Gastrointestinal upset
- Photosensitization and skin
- Pulmonary alveolitis and fibrosis
- Peripheral neuropathy.

Class IV
Verapamil, diltiazem.

Verapamil
Mechanism of Actions
- Blocks L type of Ca^{++} channels
- ↓ Ca^{++} mediated depolarization
- It has negative inotropic effect.

Uses
- PSVT, AF, AFl
- Contraindicated in AV block.

Adenosine
Mechanism of Action
It activates acetylcholine sensitive K^+ channels → hypopolarization → pacemaker depression → bradycardia, and also increased ERP → slowing of conduction.

Uses
Drug of choice in PSVT.

Adverse Drug Reactions
Transient dyspnea, fall in BP, and flushing.

Choice of Drugs for Cardiac Arrhythmias

Arrhythmia	Acute therapy (drug of choice)	Prophylaxis
PSVT	Adenosine	Digoxin/verapamil/propranolol
AFl/AF	Esmolol	Digoxin/quinidine/amiodarone
Ventricular tachycardia	Lignocaine	Amiodarone/quinidine

(AFl: atrial flutter; AF: atrial fibrilation; PSVT: paroxysmal supraventricular tachycardia)

TREATMENT OF SHOCK

- Shock—The clinical syndrome that develops when oxygen delivery is inadequate to meet the metabolic requirements of tissue due to some form of acute circulatory failure.
- *Types:*
  - Hypovolemic—Hemorrhage, severe burns, dehydration
  - Cardiogenic—Valvular heart disease, heart failure

- Obstructive—Pulmonary embolism, cardiac tamponade
- Anaphylactic—Allergy
- Septic—Bacterial toxins
- Neurogenic—Spinal anesthesia and spinal cord injury.
- *General features of shock:*
  - Hypotension (systolic BP < 100 mm Hg)
  - Tachycardia (>100)
  - Cold peripheries
  - Weak pulse
  - Low cardiac output
  - Rapid respiration
  - Drowsiness, confusion
  - Oliguria (urine output < 30 mL/min)
  - Multiorgan failure.

Note: In anaphylactic and septic shock, circulation is hyperdynamic—Warm peripheries, high bounding pulse, and high cardiac output.

Management

- Positioning of the patient (supine position, head, and chest at the same level and legs should be elevated around 10° above the horizontal level → ensures blood circulation to the brain).
- Give oxygen.
- Give positive inotropic drugs (dobutamine, dopamine).
- Maintain fluid balance (plasma expanders).
- Measure blood gases, correct if acidemia.
- Specific therapy depends on etiology.

Note: If the patient has undergone traumatic injury and is unconscious, go for ABC (airway, breathing, circulation) and CPR as per the situational demand which is also known as basic life support and to explain this is beyond the scope of this book.

Treatment of Hypovolemic Shock
- Early detection and minimizing the loss are the keys
- Restoration of fluids and plasma volume
  - Dictated by the severity of loss and patient status
  - Replacement chosen based on volume lost.

Volume Replacement
- *Crystalloids* (e.g., RL or 0.9% NS):
  - Great when loss from vomiting, intestinal obstruction, diarrhea
  - 2–3 liters can rapidly restore volume
  - It can be given while blood is cross matched.

- *Colloids* (e.g., albumin):
  - It will increase osmotic pressure, watch for pulmonary edema
  - Remain in vascular space for longer duration (several hours).
- *Blood:*
  - 500 mL whole blood increases HCT by 2-3%, 250 mL PRBC's increases HCT 3-4%
  - Increases oxygen carrying capacity
  - It is used with acute hemorrhaging.

Treatment of Cardiogenic Shock
- Increase oxygen supply to the heart—Give oxygen.
- Maximize the cardiac output
  - Maintain normal rhythm (pacing, cardioversion)
  - Medicines (dopamine, epinephrine, norepinephrine)
  - Improve myocardial contractility (give dobutamine and amrinone).
- Decrease the workload of the left ventricle:
  - Need to decrease left ventricle end diastolic pressure—Diuresis or vasodilators.

Treatment of Neurogenic Shock
- Increase vascular tone and improve cardiac output
  - Increase preload with fluids
  - Increase vascular tone: Vasopressors
  - Maintain heart rate: Treat bradycardia if symptomatic
  - Maintain adequate oxygenation
  - Initiate therapy to prevent deep vein thrombosis: Sluggish venous flow will increase risk factors.

Treatment of Anaphylactic Shock
- Goal is to stop reaction, restore vascular tone and fluid volume
- Epinephrine is used to cause vasoconstriction and reverse airway constriction
- Antihistamines used to stop the inflammatory reactions
- Bronchodilators and/or steroids to open airways
- Fluid of choice is usually ringer lactate.

Treatment of Septic Shock
- Goal is to maintain adequate tissue perfusion while providing appropriate antibiotic
  - Early detection and removal of infection
  - Watch drug levels with antibiotic's and sensitivities.

- Improve cardiac output
  - Fluid replacements
  - Inotropic agents (dobutamine)
- Provide hemodynamic support—Vasoactive drugs to increase afterload (dopamine, norepinephrine)
- Optimize oxygenation—Maintain oxygen delivery at 450-600 mL/min/m^2.

Plasma Expanders/Colloids/Colloidal Solutions
- High molecular weight substances
- Exert oncotic pressure and retain fluid in the vascular compartment.

Desirable Properties
- Should exert oncotic pressure
- Should remain in circulation
- Should be pharmacodynamically inert
- Should not be pyrogenic or antigenic
- Should not interfere with blood grouping and cross-matching
- Should be stable, easily sterilizable and cheap.

Types of Plasma Expanders (Colloids)
- Human albumin 20%
- Hydroxyethyl starch (HES, HETASTARCH)
- Dextran
- Degraded gelatin polymer
- Polyvinylpyrrolidone.

Uses of Plasma Expanders
- Substitute for plasma in the following conditions:
- Burns
- Hypovolemic and endotoxic shock
- Severe tissue damage
- In case of whole blood loss—As a temporary measure. These colloidal solutions do not have oxygen carrying capacity.

Contraindications for the Administration of Colloidal Solutions
- Severe anemia
- Cardiac failure
- Pulmonary edema
- Renal insufficiency.

CHAPTER 6

Urinary System

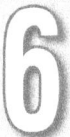

URINARY ANTISEPTICS AND DRUGS FOR URINARY TRACT INFECTION

Urinary Antiseptics
- Attain higher concentration in urine
- Nitrofurantoin and methenamine
- Nalidixic acid.

Nitrofurantoin
- Bacteriostatic may be cidal at higher concentration and in acidic urine.
- Mainly active against gram-negative organisms → reduce nitrofurantoin and generate active metabolite which damages DNA.

Pharmacokinetics
- Well absorption, rapid metabolism in liver, no therapeutic concentration in plasma and in blood; probenecid reduces tubular secretion and reduces concentration in urine.
- Contraindicated during renal failure, pregnancy, and in neonates.

Adverse Drug Reactions
- GI intolerance—Nausea, epigastric pain, and diarrhea
- Chills, fever, leukopenia (occasionally)
- Peripheral neuritis (with prolonged use)
- Hemolysis in G6PD deficiency
- Dark brown urine on exposure to air.
  Preparation: Tab 50/100 mg bid.

Use
Urinary tract infection (UTI).

Methenamine
- It decomposes slowly in acidic urine to release formaldehyde.
- pH < 5.5 is essential, mandelic acid or ascorbic acid.
  Preparation: Tab 0.5/1 g tds/qid.

Adverse Drug Reactions
- Gastritis due to release of formaldehyde in the stomach → very poor patient compliance.
- Chemical cystitis and hematuria.

Methenamine mandelate is contraindicated in renal failure and in liver failure.

Common Drugs, Used in the Treatment UTI
- Cotrimoxazole—Empirically → most pathogens including *C. trachomatis*
- Quinolones—Ciprofloxacin, norfloxacin
- Cloxacillin—Penicillinase producing organisms
- Piperacillin/carbenicillin—*Pseudomonas*
- Cephalosporins—Nosocomial *Proteus* and *Klebsiella*
- Gentamicin—Narrow margin of safety and parenteral administration limits its use.

IMPORTANT NEPHROTOXIC DRUGS

- NSAIDs—Allergic type interstitial nephritis and nephropathy, renal papillary necrosis.
- ACE inhibitors, penicillamine—Nephrotic syndrome
- Sulfonamides—Glomerulonephritis
- Aminoglycoside group of antibiotics—Tubular necrosis.

CHAPTER 7

Endocrine System

PITUITARY HORMONES

- Anterior pituitary (adenohypophysis—master endocrine gland); acidophils—growth hormone (GH), prolactin (PRL); basophils—adrenocorticotropic hormone (ACTH), thyroid-stimulating hormone (TSH), follicle-stimulating hormone (FSH) and luteinizing hormone (LH).
- Posterior pituitary—oxytocin and antidiuretic hormone (ADH).
- Intermediate lobe—melanocyte-stimulating hormone (MSH) and γ-lipoproteins.

Anterior Pituitary Hormones

Growth Hormone

Mechanism of Action

Binds to GH receptors → dimerization and activation of intracellular domain → activation of cytoplasmic JAK 2 tyrosine-protein kinase → phosphorylation of various proteins (signal transducers and activators of transcription) → synthesis of various proteins → effects.

Actions

- Indirect—Somatomedins/insulin like growth factors (IGF-1 and IGF-2); growth promotion and nitrogen retention; IGF-1 → lipogenesis and glucose uptake.
- Direct—Lipolysis, glycogenolysis, and ↓ glucose uptake → diabetogenic effects.

Regulation of Secretions

- GHRH →↑ GH
- Somatostatin; GH, IGF-1 (negative feedback) →↑ GH

Excess—Gigantism, acromegaly
Deficiency—Pituitary dwarfism.

Uses

(Human GH—Somatrem and somatropin, produced by recombinant DNA technology).

- Pituitary dwarfism—0.06-0.16 units/kg IM or SC 3 times a week up to the age of 20-25 years
- Turner's syndrome
- Renal failure
- Catabolic states—Severe burns, bedridden patients, chronic renal failure, etc.
- AIDS-related muscle wasting
  Sermorelin—Synthetic human GHRH—It is used in treatment GH deficiency
- GH antagonist—Pegvisomant (acromegaly).

Adverse Drug Reactions
- Pain at injection site
- Lipodystrophy
- Glucose intolerance
- Salt and water retention
- ↑ in intracranial pressure (ICP).

Somatostatin
- ↓ secretion of GH, TSH, PRL; also insulin and glucagon, gastrointestinal secretions.
- Constricts splanchnic, hepatic, and renal blood vessels.

Uses
- Bleeding esophageal varices and bleeding peptic ulcer (250 µg slow IV infusion over 3 minutes followed by 3 mg IV infusion over 12 h).
- Diabetic ketoacidosis (adjuvant role, ↓ glucagon, and GH).
- Acromegaly.

Octreotide
Synthetic analog of somatostatin, 40 times more potent.

Uses
- Acromegaly (preferred to somatostatin).
- Secretory diarrheas associated with carcinoid, AIDS, cancer chemotherapy.
- Bleeding esophageal varices.
- Dose—50-100 µg SC twice a day up to 500 µg TDS.

Adverse Drug Reaction
Abdominal pain, nausea, steatorrhea, gallstone.
Lanreotide—Slow release IM formulation—Once in ½ weeks in acromegaly.

Endocrine System

Prolactin (PRL)
- It causes growth and development of breast (also progesterone, estrogen).
- Promotes proliferation of ductal and acinar cells.
- Induces synthesis of milk during pregnancy.
- Induces milk secretion after parturition (↓ progesterone and estrogen → inhibition is removed).
- High level of PRL during breastfeeding → inhibitory feedback in hypothalamic-pituitary-gonadal axis → lactational amenorrhea.
- Affect immune response through action on T-lymphocytes.

Mechanism of Action

Prolactin receptor similar to GH receptor → present on cell surface → binds to PRL → transmembrane activation of cytoplasmic tyrosine protein kinase → effects.

Regulation of Secretion
- PRIH (prolactin release inhibitory hormone) → dopamine → D_2 receptor → predominant inhibition → ↓ PRL.
- Dopamine (DA) agonists—DA, bromocriptine, apomorphine → hypoprolactinemia.
- Dopamine antagonists—Chlorpromazine, haloperidol, metochlorpromide → hyperprolactinemia.
- PRF, increasing age in girls, pregnancy, suckling, stress, exertion, hypoglycemia →↑ PRL.

Hyperprolactinemia
- Galactorrhea, amenorrhea, infertility (in females)
- Loss of libido (in males).

Bromocriptine
- Synthetic ergot derivative
- Dopamine agonist (mainly via D_2 receptors)
- Partial agonist or antagonist at D_1
- Weak α adrenergic blocker.

Actions
- ↓ PRL release.
- ↑ GH release in normal individuals but ↓ from pituitary tumors causing acromegaly.
- Antiparkinsonian effect.
- Nausea and vomiting.

- Hypotension—Suppression of reflexes and peripheral α-blockade.
- ↓ GI motility.

Uses
- Hyperprolactinemia—2.5–10 mg/day.
- Acromegaly—5–20 mg/day (less effective than somatostatin and octreotide).
- Parkinsonism.
- Hepatic coma (may cause arousal).
- Suppression of lactation and breast engorgement.
- Dose: Started at low dose 1.25 mg BD then upward titration.

Adverse Drug Reactions
- Early—Nausea, vomiting, constipation, nasal blockage, postural hypotension (syncope may occur).
- Late—Behavioral alteration, mental confusion, hallucination, psychosis, abnormal movements.

Cabergoline (once/twice a week), quinagolide (once daily) → long-acting dopamine agonist used in acromegaly and hyperprolactinemia.

Gonadotropins: FSH and LH
- FSH
  - In females—Follicular growth, development of ovum, secretion of estrogens.
  - In males—Sertoli cells → Spermatogenesis.
- LH
  - In females—Preovulatory swelling of Graafian follicle → ovulation; luteinization of ruptured follicle and maintains corpus luteum; progesterone secretion.
  - In males—ICSH (interstitial cell stimulating hormone) → Leydig cells → testosterone secretion.

Mechanism of Action
FSH, LH receptors—G-protein coupled receptors →↑cAMP → gametogenesis, estrogen/testosterone synthesis.

Regulation of Secretions
- Negative feedback from testosterone and estrogen →↓ LH
- Inhibin from ovaries and testes →↓ FSH
- Dopamine →↓ LH.

Gn levels are high in menopausal women due to lack of negative feedback mechanism.

Excess—Precocious puberty and polycystic ovaries.

Deficiency—Delayed puberty, amenorrhea/sterility in females; oligozoospermia, impotence, and infertility in males.

Preparations: Given through IM route
- Menotropins—FSH + LH (obtained from urine of menopausal women)
- Urofollitropin or menotropin (pure FSH)
- Human chorionic gonadotropin (HCG) from urine of pregnant women.

Uses
- Amenorrhea and infertility
- Hypogonadotropic hypogonadism in males
- Cryptorchidism
- To aid *in vitro* fertilization.

Adverse Drug Reactions
- Ovarian hyperstimulation—Polycystic ovary, pain in lower abdomen, and even ovarian bleeding.
- Precocious puberty.
- Allergic reactions, edema, headache, and mood changes.

GnRH synthetic preparation → gonadorelin.

Long-acting/superactive GnRH agonists—Buserelin, goserelin, leuprolide, nafarelin, histerelin.

Uses
- Reversible pharmacological oophorectomy, orchiectomy in precocious puberty
- Prostatic carcinoma
- Endometriosis
- Premenopausal breast cancer
- Polycystic ovarian disease.

GnRH antagonists—Ganirelix and cetrorelix.

Thyroid Stimulating Hormone, Thyrotropin

Stimulates thyroid to synthesize and secrete thyroxine (T_4) and tri-iodothyronine (T_3).

Mechanism of Action

TSH receptor → G protein coupled receptor → ↑ cAMP → effects.

Regulation of Secretion

TRH (↑), T_3 and T_4 (negative feedback).

Endocrine System

Pathological Involvement

Myxedema (↑ TSH), Graves' disease (↓ TSH).

Use

Diagnostic → to differentiate myxedema is either due to pituitary dysfunction or primary thyroid disease. TSH injection will increase iodine uptake if thyroid is normal.

Adrenocorticotropin Hormone, Corticotropin
- Promotes steroidogenesis in adrenal cortex
- Mechanism of action-G protein coupled receptors →↑ cAMP → effects.

Regulation of Secretion

Corticotropin releasing hormone, corticosteroids (negative feedback), stressful conditions—Trauma, surgery, pain, anxiety, etc.

Pathological Involvement

Excess (from pituitary tumors)—Cushing's syndrome.

Preparation and Use
- Synthetic—Cosyntropin
- For the diagnosis of disorder of pituitary adrenal axis, cosyntropin 0.25 mg is infused IV and 24 h urine is collected. <74 micromole of 17-hydroxycorticoids → adrenal insufficiency.

Posterior Pituitary Hormones—ADH and Oxytocin

ADH
- Supraoptic nucleus
- ADH release—Osmoreceptors in hypothalamus, volume receptors in left atrium, ventricles, and pulmonary veins; plasma osmolarity.

Mechanism of Action
- ADH receptors
  - V_{1a} (blood vessels, other smooth muscles, platelets, liver, etc.)—GPCR → IP_3/DAG → Ca^{++} release → effects
  - V_{1b} (anterior pituitary)
  - V_2 receptors → GPCR → adenylyl cyclase →↑ cAMP →↑ water permeability in distal kidney tubules.
  - V_2 receptors are more sensitive to ADH.

Actions
- Kidney
    - ↑ water permeability in the collecting duct by promoting exocytosis of aquaporin-2 water channel containing vesicles (WCVs); the rate of endocytosis and degradation of WCVs is reduced.
    - Increases medullary hypertonicity by stimulating a vasopressin regulated urea transporter (VRUT) and by activating $Na^+K^+2Cl^-$ cotransporter.
    Lithium and demeclocycline partly antagonize ADH action— So they can be used in patients with inappropriate ADH secretion.
- Blood vessels: Vasopressin—Constriction of blood vessels → BP may ↑; V_2 receptor mediated vasodilation may be evident when used with V_1 antagonist or selective V_2 agonist desmopressin.
- Uterus: Contraction (via oxytocin receptors).
- CNS: Regulation of temperature, circulation, ACTH release, and in learning tasks.
- Others: Platelet aggregation, hepatic glucogenolysis, release of coagulation factor VIII, and von Willebrand factor (V_2 action).

Preparation and Dose
- Parenteral/intranasal route
- Vasopressin 10 U injection.
    Vasopressin analogs—Lypressin, terlipressin, desmopressin (selective V_2 agonist).

Uses
- Based on V_2 receptor (desmopressin; oral 0.1-0.2 mg; SC/IV—2-4 µg/day; intranasal—10-40 µg/day).
    - Diabetes insipidus—DI of pituitary origin (neurogenic)
    - Bed wetting in children and nocturia in adults
    - Hemophilia, von Willebrand disease
    - Renal concentration test—Vasopressin/desmopressin.
- Based on V_1 receptor
    - Bleeding esophageal varices—Vasopressin/terlipressin
    - Before abdominal radiography—Vasopressin/lypressin.

Adverse Drug Reactions
- Nasal irritation, congestion, rhinitis, ulceration, and epistaxis
- Belching, nausea, abdominal cramps, urge to defecate, backache in females (due to uterine contraction)

- Fluid retention and hyponatremia
- Allergic reactions.

Contraindications
- Ischemic heart disease
- Hypertension
- Chronic nephritis and psychogenic polydipsia.

Vasopressin antagonists-conivaptan ($V_{1\alpha}$ and V_2); tolvaptan (30 times V_2 than V_1).

Oxytocin
- Paraventricular nucleus; octapeptide
- Release—Coitus, parturition, suckling.

Mechanism of Action

GPCR →↑ phospholipase C → IP_3/DAG →↑ Ca^{++} → effects.

Actions
- Uterus— ↑ force and frequency of uterine contractions (with in-between relaxations).
- Breast—Contraction of myoepithelium of mammary alveoli → milk ejection reflex.
- CVS—Higher dose → vasodilatation.
- Kidney—Higher dose → ADH like effects.

Physiologic Role
- Labor
- Milk ejection reflex
- Neurotransmission—In hypothalamus and brainstem.

Preparation and Dose

IM/IV/rarely intranasal routes; 2 IU/2 mL; 5 IU/mL; 5 IU/0.5 mL injection.

Uses
- Induction of labor—5 IU is diluted in 500 mL of glucose or saline for IV infusion.
- Uterine inertia (weak uterine contractions)—Oxytocin is the drug of choice because
  - Short half-life (6 minutes)
  - Normal relaxation in-between contractions
  - No contraction of lower segment
  - Consistent augmentation of uterine contraction.

- Postpartum hemorrhage/After Cesarean section—Ergometrine is indicated. However, oxytocin is indicated in hypertensive patients.
- Breast engorgement.

Adverse Drug Reactions
- High dose (injudicious use) → strong contractions → maternal and fetal soft tissue injury, rupture of uterus, fetal asphyxia, and death.
- Water intoxication—Large dose → ADH like actions.

Contraindications
- Cephalopelvic disproportion
- Placenta previa
- Fetal distress
- Uterine scar.

INSULIN

Classification of Diabetes Mellitus
- Type 1 DM: Insulin-dependent diabetes mellitus (IDDM).
- Type 2 DM: Noninsulin-dependent diabetes mellitus (NIDDM).
- Type 3 DM: Nonpancreatic causes, drug therapy.
- Type 4 DM: Gestational diabetes mellitus.

Mechanism of Action of Insulin
- Insulin receptor—Tyrosine protein kinase receptor on the cell surface → heterotetrameric structure (2α and 2β subunits).
- Insulin binds to insulin receptor (α) → internalization of insulin-receptor complex → activation of tyrosine kinase enzyme (β) → phosphorylation of insulin receptor substrate protein (IRS1 and IRS2) → cascade of phosphorylation and dephosphorylation reactions → stimulation/inhibition of metabolic enzymes → response (RAPID EFFECTS).
- Long-term effects—Through gene transcription.

Effects of Insulin
- ↑ GLUT4
- ↓ lipolysis, ↓ proteolysis
- Regulation of glucose metabolism (↓ glycogenolysis, ↓ gluconeogenesis, ↑ glycolysis, ↑ glycogen storage)
- Regulation of gene transcription → cell proliferation and growth.

Classification of Insulin Preparations
Based on Source
- Conventional preparations
  - Pork insulin, beef insulin
  - For example regular, lente, isophane, etc.
- Purified insulin preparations
  - Single peak insulin—Proinsulin < 50–200 ppm
  - Monocomponent insulin—Proinsulin < 10 ppm.
- Human insulin
  - PRB (proinsulin recombinant bacterial) and PYR (precursor yeast recombinant)
  - More soluble—Rapid absorption*
  - Less antigenic*
  - Less insulin resistance*
  - More defined peaks*.

  *Advantages of human insulins compared to the conventional insulin preparations.
- Insulin analogs
  - Rapidly absorbed and faster acting: Insulin lispro, aspart, or glulisine.
  - Slowly released over 8–24 h: Insulin glargine and detemir.

Based on Duration of Action
- Immediate-acting (onset—0.2–0.5 h; duration—2–5 h): Insulin lispro, aspart, or glulisine (insulin analogs).
- Short-acting (onset 0.5–1 h; duration 6–8 h): Regular (soluble) insulin.
- Intermediate-acting (onset 1–2 h; duration 20–24 h): Insulin zinc suspension or lente, NPH (neutral protamine Hagedorn), isophane insulin.
- Long-acting (onset 4–6 h; duration 24–36 h)
  - Protamine zinc insulin, ultralente
  - Insulin glargine and insulin detemir (insulin analogs).

Insulin Delivery System
- Disposable insulin syringe
- Portable pen injector
- Continuous subcutaneous insulin infusion (CSII):
  - Regular insulin, insulin lispro, aspart, and glulisine
  - Abdomen, flanks, thigh
  - Physiological, excellent glycemic control, expensive.

- Inhaled insulin: To control meal time hyperglycemia.
- Implantable pump and external artificial pancreas.

Adverse Effects of Insulin
- Hypoglycemia—Tachycardia, confusion, vertigo, and diaphoresis
- Lipodystrophy (minimal or absent with newer preparation)
- Hypersensitivity (rare with newer preparation)
- Edema.

ORAL ANTIDIABETIC AGENTS
Classification of Oral Antidiabetic Agents
- Insulin secretion enhancers
    - Sulfonylureas (K_{ATP} channel blockers in pancreatic beta cells):
        - *First generation*—Tolbutamide, chlorpropamide
        - *Second generation*—Glibenclamide, glipizide, gliclazide, glimepiride
    - Meglitinide analog: Repaglinide; nateglinide (not meglitinide analog)
    - Incretin modulators
        - *Glucagon-like peptide-1 (GLP-1) receptor agonists*: Exenatide, liraglutide
        - *Dipeptidyl peptidase-IV inhibitors*: Sitagliptin, vildagliptin, saxagliptin.
- Insulin resistance inhibitors
    - Biguanides [Adenosine monophosphate dependent protein kinase (AMP-K) activator]: Metformin
    - Thiazolidinediones [Activators of peroxisome proliferator-activated receptor γ (PPARγ)]: Pioglitazone, rosiglitazone.
- Miscellaneous agents
    - Alpha-glucosidase inhibitors: Acarbose, miglitol, voglibose
    - Sodium glucose co-transport-2 (SGLT-2) inhibitor: Canagliflozin, dapagliflozin, empagliflozin
- Amylin analog: Pramlintide
- Dopamine D_2 receptor agonist: Bromocriptine
- Bile acid sequestrant: Colesevelam.

Mechanism of Action of Important Oral Antidiabetic Agents
Sulfonylureas
Bind to sulfonylurea receptors in pancreatic beta cells → block ATP-sensitive potassium channels → depolarization → influx of calcium → release of insulin.

Meglitinide Analog: Repaglinide
Similar to sulfonylureas; blocks ATP sensitive K⁺ channels → depolarization → insulin release.

Biguanides: Metformin (Phenformin Outdated, Because of its Lactic Acidosis)
- ↓ Gluconeogenesis and glycogenolysis → ↓ hepatic glucose output → ↓ blood glucose
- Metformin is euglycemic drug (does not cause hypoglycemia).

Glucagon-like Peptide-1 (GLP-1) Receptor Agonist: Exenatide, Liraglutide
GLP-1→ incretin (gut hormone) released by gut → ↑ insulin, ↓ glucagon, and gastric emptying. So GLP-1 agonists act in a similar manner.

Dipeptidyl Peptidase-4 Inhibitors: Sitagliptin, Linagliptin, Saxagliptin
↑GLP-1 (mainly) also ↑GIP (glucose-dependent insulinotropic peptide) → ↑ postprandial insulin release and ↓ glucagon → ↓ blood glucose.

α-Glucosidase Inhibitor—Acarbose
↓ Reduce postprandial blood glucose by inhibiting α-glucosidase (α-glucosidase breaks down poly and disaccharides) →↓ intestinal absorption of glucose.

Sodium Glucose Cotransporter-2 (SGLT-2) Inhibitor—Canagliflozin, Dapagliflozin, Empagliflozin
↓ SGLT-2 (sodium glucose transporter-2: Responsible for absorption of 90% of filtered glucose) in renal proximal tubules → glycosuria → ↓ blood glucose.

Amylin Analog—Pramlintide
↓ Glucagon, ↓ gastric emptying, ↓ glucose absorption, and promotes satiety.

Indications of Oral Antidiabetic Agents
Oral antidiabetic agents are prescribed in type 2 DM in the following conditions:
- Age > 40 years at onset of disease
- Obesity
- Duration— <5 years
- FBG < 200 mg/dL

- Insulin requirement < 40 U/day
- No complications when starting treatment.

Important Side Effects of Oral Antidiabetics
- *Sulfonylureas:* Hypoglycemia, weight gain, drug-drug interactions
- *Metformin:* Lactic acidosis (check renal function test, contraindicated in severe renal impairment)
- *Thiazolidinediones (pioglitazone, rosiglitazone):* Fluid retention, aggravation of congestive heart failure; hepatotoxicity
- *Acarbose:* Flatulence, diarrhea (due to undigested carbohydrates)
- *Sodium glucose co-transport-2 (SGLT-2) inhibitor (canagliflozin and others):* Urinary and genital infections (due to ↑ glucose in urine).

PHARMACOLOGY OF CORTICOSTEROIDS

Classifications

Based on Duration of Action and Anti-Inflammatory Potency
Relative Activity of Systemic Corticosteroids

		Compound	Glucocorticoids	Mineralocorticoids	Equiv. dose (anti-inflammatory)
Glucocorticoids	Short acting (biological) (t½ < 2 h)	Hydrocortisone (cortisol)	1	1	20 mg
		Cortisone	0.8	0.8	25 mg
	Intermediate acting, (biological) (t½ 12–36 h)	Prednisolone	4	0.8	5 mg
		Methyl prednisolone	5	0.5	4 mg
		Triamcinolone	5	0	4 mg
	Long acting (Biological) (t½ > 36 h)	Paramethasone	10	0	2 mg
		Dexamethasone	25	0	0.75 mg
		Betamethasone	25	0	0.75 mg
Mineralocorticoids					Equiv. salt retaining dose
		Desoxycorticosterone acetate (DOCA)	0	100	2.5 mg (sublingual)
		Fludrocortisone	10	150	0.2 mg
		Aldosterone	0.3	3000	not used clinically

Based on Mode of Administration
- Systemic—Hydrocortisone, prednisolone, etc.
- Topical—Alclometasone, clobetasol, fluocinolone
- Inhalational—Budesonide, fluticasone (also topical), beclomethasone (also topical)
- Ophthalmic—Fluorometholone, medrysone.

Uses
- Replacement therapy
    - Acute adrenal insufficiency—Hydrocortisone.
    - Chronic adrenal insufficiency (Addison's disease)—Hydrocortisone ± fludrocortisone.
    - Congenital adrenal hyperplasia (adrenogenital syndrome)—Hydrocortisone.
- Diagnostic
    - Dexamethasone suppression test—1 mg oral at 11 PM and take plasma sample the following morning to check cortisol level; < 3 µg/dL → normal, >5 µg/dL → Cushing syndrome.
- Pharmacotherapy
- Allergic reactions: Angioneurotic edema, contact dermatitis, and urticaria.
- Collagen vascular diseases: Rheumatoid arthritis, polymyositis, and giant cell arthritis.
- Eye diseases: Acute uveitis and allergic conjunctivitis.
- Gastrointestinal disease: Inflammatory bowel disease.
- Hematological disorders: Hemolytic anemia, leukemia, idiopathic thrombocytopenic purpura, and multiple myeloma.
- Systemic inflammation: Acute respiratory distress syndrome.
- Inflammatory conditions of bones and joints: Arthritis, bursitis, and tenosynovitis.
- Neurological disorders: Cerebral edema and multiple sclerosis.
- Organ transplants: Prevention and treatment of rejection.
- Pulmonary diseases: Aspiration pneumonia, bronchial asthma, and infant respiratory distress syndrome (for fetal lung maturation).
- Renal disorder: Nephrotic syndrome.
- Skin diseases: Atopic dermatitis, dermatoses, pemphigus, and seborrheic dermatitis.
- Infections: Tubercular meningitis, lepra reactions, and *Pneumocystis jiroveci* pneumonia in AIDS patients.

- Miscellaneous
  - Autoimmune diseases—Myasthenia gravis, and autoimmune hemolytic anemia.
  - Shock, hypercalcemia, mountain sickness, and lymphoma.

Adverse Effects
- Due to mineralocorticoid actions: Sodium and water retention, edema, hypertension, hypokalemia, alkalosis.
- Due to glucocorticoid actions
  - Cushing's habitus—Moon face, narrow mouth, buffalo hump, obesity with thin limbs
  - Muscular weakness
  - Fragile/thin skin, easy bruising
  - Opportunistic infections
  - Delayed healing, peptic ulcer
  - Osteoporosis: Compression/spontaneous fracture, avascular necrosis of head of femur
  - Cataract, glaucoma
  - Growth retardation, fetal abnormalities (cleft palate,↓ intrauterine growth)
  - Psychiatric problems: Manic psychosis.
- HPA axis (hypothalamus-pituitary-adrenal axis) suppression
  - 20 mg hydrocortisone or equivalent/day for 2 weeks, taper the doses (do not stop abruptly)
  - 20 mg hydrocortisone or equivalent/day for 2 weeks within 2 years of therapy → suspect HPA suppression and give supplemental doses.
- Rules to minimize HPA suppression—5S
  - Shorter acting
  - Shortest period
  - Single dose in morning
  - Switch to alternate day therapy
  - Systemic therapy—Limit/local.

Note: These 5S should be practiced as far as possible.

THYROID HORMONES AND ANTITHYROID DRUGS
Thyroid Hormones
Preparations
- Natural: Desiccated thyroid (animal origin).
- Synthetic

- L-thyroxine (T_4)
- Liothyronine (T_3)
- Liotrix ($T_4 + T_3$).
- L-thyroxine is preferred: 4M—Money, multiple dose, monitoring (difficult), myocardium (cardiac toxicity)—More with T_3.

Indications
- For replacement therapy
- For TSH suppression therapy
- Replacement therapy
  - Cretinism
  - Adult hypothyroidism
  - Myxedema coma.
- Suppression therapy
  - Nontoxic goiter/endemic goiter (also a replacement of therapy)
  - Thyroid nodule (functioning— ↑ TSH)
  - Papillary carcinoma of thyroid (↑ TSH, and nonresectable).

Antithyroid Drugs
Classifications
- Synthesis inhibitors/thioamides
  - Propylthiouracil (PTU)
  - Methimazole
  - Carbimazole.
- Inhibit iodine trapping (anion inhibitors)
  - Thiocyanates (SCN^-)
  - Perchlorates (ClO^{-4})
  - Pertechnetate (TcO^{-4}).
- Inhibit hormone release
  - Iodine, iodides of Na and K, Lugol's iodine (5% iodine in 10% KI).
- Destroy thyroid tissue: Radioactive iodine (^{131}I).
- Iodinated contrast media: Diatrizoate, iohexol.

Adjuvant
- β-blocker—Propranolol, esmolol (to ↓ sympathetic over activity)
- Calcium channel blocker—Diltiazem, verapamil (to ↓ palpitation if beta blockers are contraindicated)
- Corticosteroids—Hydrocortisone.

Sites of Action of Antithyroid Drugs

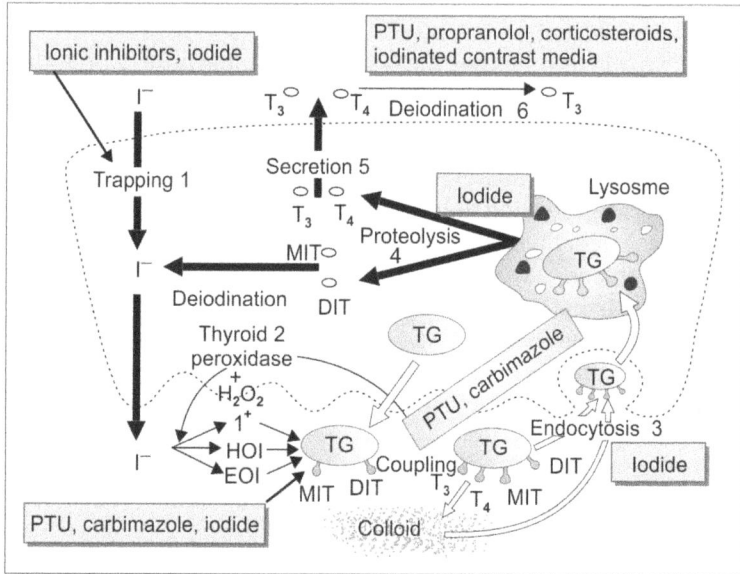

(PTU: propylthiouracil; TG: thyroglobulin; EOI: enzyme linked hypoiodate; DIT: diiodotyrosine; MIT: monoiodotyrosine; HOI: hypoiodous acid)

DRUGS ACTING ON UTERINE MUSCULATURE (OXYTOCICS AND TOCOLYTICS)

- Uterine stimulants (oxytocics, abortifacients)
- Uterine relaxants (tocolytics).

Uterine Stimulants

- Hormone—Oxytocin
- Ergot alkaloids—Ergometrine, methylergometrine
- Prostaglandins—$PGE_{2\alpha}$, $PGF_{2\alpha}$, misoprostol
- Others—Ethacridine, quinine.

Uses

- Induction of labor
- Uterine inertia
- Postpartum hemorrhage
- Breast engorgement.

Side Effects
- Maternal and fetal soft tissue injury, fetal asphyxia
- Water intoxication
- Increase in BP.

Uterine Relaxants
- Adrenergic agonists (β_2-selective) ritodrine, salbutamol
- Magnesium sulfate
- Calcium channel blockers
- Prostaglandin synthesis inhibitors, ethyl alcohol, progesterone, nitrites.

Uses
- To delay labor
- To arrest threatened abortion
- Dysmenorrhea
- Premature labor.

Side Effects
β_2-selective
- Cardiovascular—Arrhythmias
- Metabolic—Hyperglycemia
- Anxiety, headache.

Magnesium Sulfate
- Cardiac arrhythmias, muscular paralysis
- CNS and respiratory depression.

Calcium Channel Blockers
Tachycardia and hypotension.

PHARMACOLOGY OF MALE AND FEMALE SEX HORMONES

Male Sex Hormones
- Androgens
    - Natural androgens
        - Testosterone
        - Dehydroepiandrosterone
        - Androstenedione.
    - Synthetic androgens
        - Methyltestosterone
        - Fluoxymesterone

- Testosterone undecanoate
- Mesterolone.

Pharmacokinetics
- Testosterone—Inactive orally due to high first pass metabolism 98% is bound to plasma protein.
- Mainly excreted through kidney.

Mechanism of Action
Testosterone → (by 5 α-reductase) → dihydrotestosterone (in some tissues, in others testosterone itself binds to the nuclear receptors) → binds with nuclear receptor → regulates protein synthesis → modulation of the biological functions.

Uses
- Testicular failure
- Hypopituitarism
- AIDS-related muscle wasting
- Hereditary angioneurotic edema.

Side Effects
- Acne
- Priapism
- Edema
- Cholestatic jaundice
- Hepatic carcinoma
- Gynecomastia
- Virilization and menstrual irregularities in woman.

Female Sex Hormones
- Estrogens
- Progesterones
- Natural estrogens—Estradiol
- Synthetic estrogens steroidal—Ethylestradiol, mestranol non-steroidal-diethylstilbestrol (stilbestrol) hexesterol.

Estrogens
Pharmacokinetics
- Synthetic estrogens → well-absorbed orally and transdermally.
- Natural estrogen → inactive orally (high first pass metabolism).
- High plasma protein binding.
- Excreted in urine and bile.

Mechanism of Action
Estrogen → nuclear receptor → protein synthesis → regulation of functions.

Uses
- Hormone replacement therapy
- Senile vaginitis
- Delayed puberty in girls
- Others—Dysmenorrhea, acne, hirsutism, dysfunctional uterine bleeding, carcinoma prostate.

Side Effects
- Venous thromboembolism
- Gallstones
- Endometrial carcinoma
- Breast cancer
- Suppression of libido, gynecomastia, and feminization of males
- Progestins
- Natural progestin—Progesterone
- Synthetic progestin—Medroxyprogesterone acetate, norgestrel.

Progesterones

Pharmacokinetics
Progesterone is inactive orally. Synthetic progestins are orally active. Metabolic products are excreted in the urine.

Mechanism of Action
Binds to nuclear receptor which results in the synthesis of proteins → regulation of functions.

Uses
- As contraceptive
- Hormone replacement therapy
- Endometriosis
- Premenstrual tension
- Threatened/habitual abortion
- Endometrial carcinoma.

Side Effects
- Breast engorgement
- Headache
- Rise in body temperature
- Mood swings

- Irregular bleeding
- Blood sugar may rise
- Some preparations are atherogenic (norgestrel).

METHODS OF CONTRACEPTION

Classifications
- Natural method
  - Abstinence
  - Outer course
  - Lactation amenorrhea method.
- Barrier method
  - Condoms (male and female)
  - Cervical cap
  - Cervical diaphragm
- Spermicidal
- Intrauterine device (IUD)
- Hormonal contraception
  - Female
    - Oral (combined pill, phasic pill, mini pill, postcoital/emergency)
    - Injectable
    - Implant
  - Male
- Sterilization
  - Male
    - Vasectomy
  - Female
    - Tubal ligation; mini-laparotomy incision, laparoscopically, or transcervically
    - Hysterectomy

Natural Method
- Abstinence
  - 0% failure rate
  - Ideal for adolescents at high risk for pregnancy and STDs including HIV.
- Outer course: Sexual activity without penetration.
- Lactation amenorrhea method (LAM)
  - Mechanism: Suckling causes increased PRL
  - Inhibits estrogen production and ovulation

- 2% failure rate in first 6 months, 33–45% ovulate during first 3 months.

Barrier Methods
- Condoms—Male
  - Sheaths of latex or polyurethane that may or may not have spermicide.
  - Failure rate is 15%.
- Condoms—Female
  - Disposable single use polyurethane sheath placed in vagina.
  - Flexible movable inner ring at closed end used to insert into vagina.
  - Failure rate is 21%.
- Cervical cap
  - Thimble-shaped latex rubber device which has an inner ring that provides suction to keep cap on the cervix.
  - Spermicide is placed inside the cap before being placed on the cervix to kill sperm.
  - Four sizes: 22, 25, 28, 31 mm.
  - It can be placed 6 h prior to intercourse.
  - It can remain in vagina up to 48 h for multiple acts of intercourse.
- Cervical diaphragm
  - Latex rubber dome-shaped device that covers the cervix.
  - Failure rate: 16%.

Spermicidal
- Most common is nonoxynol-9
- Available in creams, films, foams, and gels
- Suppositories, sponges, and tablets
- Best when used with barrier methods
- 29% failure rate when used alone.

Intrauterine Device
- Copper and plastic (Copper T-380A): Effective for 10 years
- Plastic and progesterone [intrauterine device (IUD)] 1 year
- 90–96% effectively in use
- Increased risk of PID/perforation/hemorrhage.

Hormonal Contraception
Mechanism of Action
- ↓ Gonadotropins (Gn-FSH, LH) secretion (estrogen and progestin).

- Thick cervical mucous → not favorable for sperm penetration (progestin).
- Hyperproliferative/hypersecretory, atrophic endometrium → Failure of implantation (minipill and postcoital pill).
- Uterine tubal contraction/interfere with implantation/dislodge blastocyst (postcoital pill).

Female
- Oral—Combined pill, phasic pill, mini pill, postcoital/emergency
  - Combined pill
    - Most efficacious, most popular
    - Failure rate is 0.1%
    - Levonorgestrel 0.25 mg and ethinyl estradiol 50 μg
    - Taken daily for 21 days (start on 5th day of menstruation), 7 days gap.
  - Phasic pill-mono/bi/triphasic
    - Estrogen is varied slightly (30–40 μg), amount of progestin is low in first phase, progressively higher in second and third phases (100–150 μg or 50, 75, and 125 μg).
  - Mini pill
    - Progestin only
    - Taken daily without any gap
    - Failure rate is 20–30%.
  - Centchroman—Developed in India: Anti-implantation agent.
  - Postcoital/emergency contraception
    - Levonorgestrel 0.5 mg + ethinyl estradiol 0.1 mg, twice with 12 h gap within 72 h—Yuzpe method.
    - Levonorgestrel alone 0.75 mg, twice with 12 h gap within 72 h.
    - Mifepristone 600 mg single dose within 72 h.
- Injectable
  - DMPA (depomedroxyprogesterone) 150 mg tri-monthly—Sangini Sui.
  - Norethindrone enanthate 200 mg/2 months.
- Implant
  - Copper IUD—Place within 5 days of unprotected coitus.
  - This is usually given to women who plan to use the IUD for long-term birth control.
  - Interferes with implantation after fertilization.
  - 6 × 36 mg levonorgestrel SC—Norplant
  - Effective for 5 years.

Side Effects
- Nausea, vomiting, headache (↑ migraine).
- Breakthrough bleedings/spotting, breast discomfort.
- Weight gain, chloasma, mood swings, carbohydrate intolerance.
- Leg vein, pulmonary, coronary, and cerebral thrombosis (↑ myocardial ischemia, stroke).
- ↑ blood pressure, genital carcinoma/gallstones/hepatoma.

Contraindications
Absolute
- Thromboembolic disorders (history of stroke, myocardial infarction)
- Hypertension
- History of jaundice
- Suspected breast/genital malignancy.

Relative
- Diabetes mellitus, obesity, smoking
- Amoxicillin/ampicillin therapy
- Undiagnosed vaginal bleeding
- >35 years, mentally ill, migraine.

Practical Considerations
- Return of fertility occurs within 1–2 months after discontinuation, initial 2–3 cycle-chances of multiple pregnancy.
- If one tab is missed, take two tabs next day. If more than two doses are missed, then discontinue or adopt alternative method.
- If pregnancy occurs, termination should be done.
- Obese may require higher ethinyl estradiol (50 μg).

Male contraception
- Complete suppression of spermatogenesis (takes 64 days)—Difficult.
- Gonadotropin suppression—Suppression of testosterone—Many adverse drug reactions.
- Men do not get pregnant—Compliance poor.
- Antiandrogens, estrogen/progesterone, superactive GnRH analog →↓ Gn.
- Gossypol →↓ spermatogenesis.

Sterilization
Male—Vasectomy
- Vas deferens are cut and sealed ↓ LA
- No passage of sperm into seminal fluid

- Cheaper than female sterilization
- Failure rate is <0.15%
- Use other contraceptive methods until complete azoospermia → usually 12 weeks or 10-20 ejaculations
- Orgasm is not affected.

Female—Tubal ligations
- Cut and seal the fallopian tubes
- Interrupt the patency of fallopian tubes
- Thereby preventing fertilization
- Failure rate depends on method used; ranges from 0.8 to 3.7%
- It may be performed through a mini-laparotomy incision, laparoscopically, or transcervically.
- Hysterectomy: Removal of the uterus.

TREATMENT OF SEXUALLY TRANSMITTED DISEASES
Sexually Transmitted Diseases
- Infections that can be transferred from one person to another through sexual contact.
- Almost 10% of infections which cause serious disease or present difficulty in diagnosis are almost sexually transmitted.
- The United States has the highest rates of sexually transmitted diseases (STDs or STIs), an estimated 15.3 million new cases/year.
- Females > males.

Complications
- Cervical cancer
- Liver disease
- Pelvic inflammatory disease, infertility (male and female)
- Pregnancy problems.

Treatment
- The treatment depends on the types of STD
- For some STDs, curative treatment
- For other STDs, symptomatic treatment.

Genital Herpes
- Analgesic agent such as 2% lignocaine
- Acyclovir 3% as an ointment
- Acyclovir 200 mg 4 hourly for 5 days
- Betadine to control secondary infections.

Condyloma Accuminata (Veneral/Genital Wart)
- 20% podophyllin
- Electrocautery
- Laser surgery
- Surgical excision.

Molluscum Contagiosum
- Phenol 80%
- Diathermy and cryosurgery.

Gonorrhea
- Ceftriaxone 250 mg IM/cefuroxime 250 mg IM + probenecid 1 g oral
- Procaine penicillin 4.8 MU IM + probenecid 1 g
- Amoxicillin 3 g oral/ampicillin 3.5 g oral + probenecid 1 g.

Alternatives
Ciprofloxacin 250–500 mg/ofloxacin 200–400 mg single dose.

Syphilis
- Early (primary, secondary, and late < 1 year)
    - Benzathine penicillin 2.4 MU IM 1–3 weekly
    - Jarisch-Herxheimer reaction-prednisolone 5 mg qid one day before and 2 days after.

  Alternatives
    - Erythromycin 500 mg qid, doxycycline 100 mg bid for 10–15 days.
- Late syphilis (>1 year)
    - Benzathine penicillin 2.4 MU IM weekly for 4 weeks.

  Alternatives
    - Doxycycline or erythromycin for 30 days.

HIV and AIDs
Antiretroviral Drugs
- Nucleoside reverse transcriptase (RT) inhibitors—Zidovudine, didanosine, lamivudine, stavudine
- Nucleotide RT inhibitor—Tenofovir
- Nonnucleoside RT inhibitors—Delavirdine, nevirapine
- Protease inhibitors—Ritonavir, saquinavir
- Fusion/entry inhibitor—Enfuvirtide.

Hepatitis B
- Symptomatic treatment
- Interferon α-(IFN-α) inhibits viral replication (penetration, synthesis, assembly)
- Liver transplant
- Hepatitis B vaccine (for prevention).

Chlamydia Trachomatis (Silent Disease)
- Nonspecific urethritis: Azithromycin 1 g single dose or doxycycline 100 mg for 7 days.
- Lymphogranuloma venereum: Doxycycline 100 mg for 2 weeks.

Granuloma Inguinale
Tetracycline 500 mg qid for 10 days or doxycycline 100 mg bid for 3 weeks.

Chancroid
Ceftriaxone 250 mg IM single dose or ciprofloxacin 500 mg bid for 3 days.

Trichomonas Vaginalis
- Metronidazole 2 g single dose or 400 mg tds for 7 days.
- Clotrimazole 100 mg intravaginal
- Tinidazole 2 g single dose.

Treat the male partner also if recurrent.

Bacterial Vaginosis (Bacterial Vaginitis, Anaerobic Vaginosis)
- Metronidazole 2 g oral single dose
- Clindamycin—Topical application.

Candida Vaginalis
- Clotrimazole—Use as pessaries or vaginal tablets or cream
- Fluconazole 150 mg single dose.

Prevention
- Abstinence
- Be faithful to the partner
- Use of condoms
- Regular pelvic examinations
- Vaccination against hepatitis B
- Maintenance of proper genital hygiene.

ANABOLIC STEROIDS
- Ratio of androgenic:anabolic activity of testosterone = 1:1.
- Anabolic steroids have ratios between 1:3 and 1:10.
- Increase bone density, muscle mass, heme synthesis, sense of well-being, and decrease proteolysis.
- These are included in "Dope test" in sports.
- Examples—Methandienone, nandrolone, oxymetholone, and stanozolol.
- These are most commonly abused by athletes to increase strength and performance.

Uses
- After trauma, surgery (to ↓ protein loss)
- AIDS patients (to ↓ muscle wasting)
- Hereditary angioneurotic edema (oxymetholone and stanozolol →↑ complement Cl^- esterase inhibitor).

Side Effects
- In males—Testicular atrophy, sterility, and gynecomastia
- In females—Inhibition of ovulation, hirsutism, deepening of voice, frontal alopecia, and acne.

CALCIFICATION AND BONE TURNOVER: PARATHORMONE (PARATHYROID HORMONE), VITAMIN D, AND CALCITONIN
- Calcification—Incorporation of Ca^{++} ions as a crystalline hydroxyapatite on organic bone matrix osteoid.
- Remodeling—Resorption and new bone formation.
- Osteoblast, osteoclast.

Factors Affecting Bone Turnover
- Factors that increase bone resorption
    - Corticosteroids
    - Parathormone
    - Hypervitaminosis D
    - PGE_2
    - IL 1 and 6
    - Alcoholism
    - Loop diuretic agents.
- Factors that decrease bone resorption
    - Estrogens and androgens
    - Calcitonin

- Growth hormone
- Bisphosphonates (etidronate, pamidronate, alendronate)
- Fluoride
- Thiazide diuretics.
- Parathormone (parathyroid hormone)
  - Secretion is controlled by blood Ca^{++} level
  - The higher the level → the lesser the secretion and vice versa.

Effects

- Bone—Parathyroid hormone (PTH) ↑ bone resorption→↑ blood Ca^{++} level
- Kidney—It increases reabsorption of Ca^{++} in distal tubule
- Intestine—It helps in formation of calcitriol which in turn enhances Ca^{++} absorption
- Hypoparathyroidism—Hypocalcemia, tetany, convulsions, laryngospasm, paresthesia
- Hyperparathyroidism—Hypercalcemia, decalcification → bone deformities and fractures (osteitis fibrosa generalisata), renal stone, muscle weakness.

Calcitonin

- Secreted by parafollicular cells (C cells) of thyroid gland
- Hypocalcemic hormone
- Secretion is dependent on the plasma Ca^{++} level.

Effects

- Opposite of PTH **(Figs. 7.1 and 7.2)**
- Bone—Decreases bone resorption
- Kidney—Inhibits Ca^{++} and phosphate reabsorption in proximal tubules.

Uses

- Hypercalcemic states (hyperparathyroidism, hypervitaminosis D)
- Postmenopausal osteoporosis
- Paget's disease (osteitis deformans).

Parathyroid hormone acts on osteoblasts and indirectly activates osteoclasts, as well as recruits osteoclast precursors in bone remodeling units. Calcitriol promotes differentiation of osteoclast precursors. Facilitated by PTH calcitriol increases osteoblast

Endocrine System

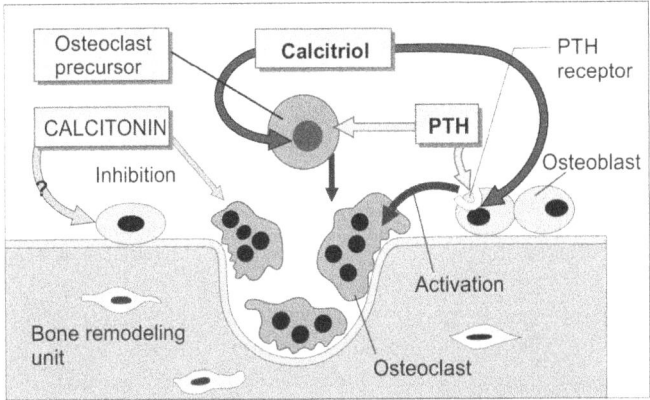

Fig. 7.1: Hormonal regulation of bone remodeling units.

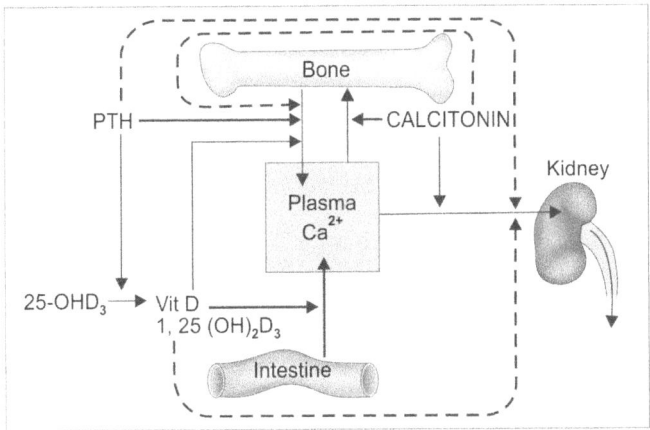

Fig. 7.2: Regulation of plasma level of calcium.

mediated activation of osteoclasts. Calcitonin inhibits osteoclastic activity and probably increases osteoblastic activity.
→ Stimulation, → inhibition; bold arrow—major action. PTH—parathormone; 25-OHD$_3$—calcifediol; 1,25 (OH)$_2$D$_3$—calcitriol

Vitamin D

- Vitamin D → vitamin D$_3$ (cholecalciferol)—In skin; vitamin D$_2$ calciferol—In irradiated food
- Active form—Calcitriol (1,25-dihydroxyvitamin D).

Effects
- Intestine—↑ Ca^{++} and phosphate absorption.
- Bone—It helps in bone mineralization by maintaining normal plasma Ca^{++} and phosphate levels.
- Kidney—It increases proximal tubular reabsorption of Ca^{++} and phosphate.

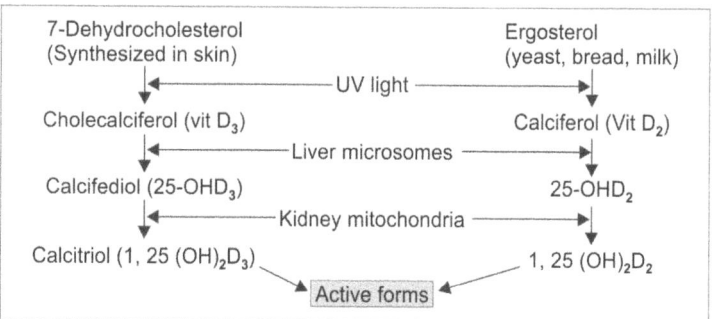

- Deficiency—(high levels of PTH; increased bone resorption, bones fail to mineralize normally)
  - Rickets in children
  - Osteomalacia in adults.

Preparations
- Calciferol (ergocalciferol, vitamin D_2)
- Cholecalciferol (vitamin D_3)
- Calcitriol
- Alfacalcidol (1α-OHD).

Uses
- Prophylaxis and treatment of nutritional vitamin deficiency
- Rickets
- Senile or postmenopausal osteoporosis
- Hypoparathyroidism.

CHAPTER 8

Gastrointestinal and Hepatobiliary System

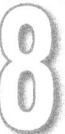

DRUGS USED IN PEPTIC ULCER

Peptic Ulcer
- Gastric/duodenal
- Mucosal defensive factors—Mucus, mucosal blood flow, formation of HCO^-_3 and PGE_2 and PGI_2
- Aggressive factors—Acid, pepsin, NSAIDs, *Helicobacter pylori*.

Imbalance between aggressive factors (more active) and defensive factors (less active) → peptic ulcer formation, so during treatment defensive factors should be increased or potenciated and aggressive factors should be inhibited or minimized.

Classifications
- Drugs which reduce gastric acid secretion
    - H_2 receptor antagonists (H_2 antihistaminics)—Cimetidine, ranitidine, famotidine, roxatidine, loratadine
    - Proton-pump inhibitors—Omeprazole, lansoprazole, pantoprazole, rabeprazole
    - Anticholinergics—Propantheline, pirenzepine, telenzepine
    - Prostaglandin analogs—Misoprostol (PGE_1), enprostil (PGE_2), rioprostil (PGE_1).
- Drugs which neutralize gastric acid (antacids)
    - Systemic—Sodium bicarbonate
    - Nonsystemic—aluminum hydroxide, aluminum phosphate, magnesium trisilicate, magaldrate, magnesium hydroxide, and calcium carbonate.
- Ulcer protective—Sucralfate, colloidal bismuth subcitrate.
- Ulcer healing drugs—Carbenoxolone sodium.
- Anti-*Helicobacter pylori* drugs (used in combination) amoxicillin, clarithromycin, metronidazole, tinidazole, tetracycline.

Uses of Antiulcer Medicines
- Duodenal ulcer
- Gastric ulcer
- Stress ulcer and gastritis
- Zollinger-Ellison syndrome (gastric hypersecretory state)
- To prevent aspiration pneumonia (before major surgery)
- Gastroesophageal reflux disease.

Anti-Helicobacter *Pylori* Regimen
- *H. pylori*—Gram-negative bacteria
- High urease activity (urea → ammonia → neutralizes gastric HCl around the bacteria; negative feedback → more gastrin; proteases and lipases → chronic inflammation and ulcer)
- Commensal in 20–70% of normal individuals
- Associated with 90% of gastric and duodenal ulcers
- Lansoprazole 30 mg BD + amoxicillin 1000 mg BD + clarithromycin 500 mg BD for 2 weeks → 86–92% eradication.

EMETICS AND ANTIEMETICS
Vomiting
- Expulsion of gastric contents through mouth due to mass antiperistalsis
- Nausea—Uneasy feeling in anticipation of vomiting
- Protective mechanism but can be a nuisance
- Caused by diseases and drugs
- Also occurs in:
  - Early pregnancy (first trimester)
  - Motion/sea sickness
  - Radiation, postoperative, and cancer chemotherapy.

Emetics
- Drugs used to induce vomiting
- Apomorphine—It acts on chemoreceptor trigger zone (CTZ) (D_2 agonism), IM/SC, acts within 5 min
- Ipecacuanha—It acts by irritating gastric mucosa and also via CTZ, oral route, acts within 15 min.

Antiemetics
Drugs to prevent or suppress vomiting.

Classifications
- Anticholinergics—Hyoscine, dicyclomine, scopolamine
- H_1 antihistaminics—Promethazine, diphenhydramine, dimenhydrinate, cyclizine, meclizine, doxylamine, cinnarizine
- Neuroleptics—Chlorpromazine, prochlorperazine, haloperidol
- Prokinetic agents—Metoclopramide, domperidone, cisapride, mosapride, renzapride, itopride
- $5\text{-}HT_3$ antagonists—Ondansetron, granisetron
- Adjuvant antiemetics—Dexamethasone, benzodiazepines (BZDs), cannabinoids (nabilone, dronabinol).

Choices of Drugs
- Motion sickness
  - Hyoscine/scopolamine
  - Diphenhydramine dimenhydrinate, cyclizine, meclizine, promethazine, cinnarizine.
- Morning sickness (for hyperemesis gravidarum)
  - Dicyclomine
  - Doxylamine, cyclizine, meclizine
  - Pyridoxine (vitamin B_6).
- Chemotherapy-induced vomiting/emesis (CIE)
  - $5\text{-}HT_3$ receptor antagonists—Ondansetron, granisetron, dolasetron
  - Prochlorperazine, metoclopramide, domperidone
  - Dexamethasone, diazepam.
- Postoperative vomiting
  - Metoclopramide, ondansetron, prochlorperazine.

DRUGS USED IN CONSTIPATION AND DIARRHEA

Constipation
Delayed passage of feces through the intestine, evacuation is often associated with straining leading to sensation of incomplete evacuation.

Causes
- Functional—Bedridden patients, dietary habits, and sedentary lifestyle
- GI diseases—Colon cancer, stricture, and irritable bowel syndrome
- Systemic diseases—Hypothyroidism

- Drugs—Opioids, Ca^{++} channel blocker, anticholinergics, laxative abuse.

Treatment of Constipations
- Nonpharmacological: Fiber diet (grain, vegetables, fruits), regular exercise, sufficient water intake, and not neglecting nature's call.
- Pharmacological.

Drugs for Constipation
- Aperients < Laxatives < Emollients < Purgatives < Cathartics
- Purgative in smaller dose = Laxative or vice versa
- Laxatives result in elimination of semisolid stool
- Purgatives result in more watery evacuation.

Classifications
- Bulk forming (1-3 days)
    - Dietary fibers—Bran, ispaghula husk
    - Methylcellulose.
- Stool softeners (1-3 days)
    - Docusate sodium
    - Liquid paraffin.
- Stimulant purgatives (6-8 hours)
    - Phenolphthalein
    - Bisacodyl
    - Senna.
- Osmotic purgatives (1-3 hours)
    - Mg salts—$MgSO_4$ and $Mg(OH)_2$
    - Na+ salts—Sulfate and phosphate
    - Lactulose (1-3 days)
    - Polyethylene glycol (PEG).
- Chloride channel opener
    - Lubiprostone (PGE1 analog)

Uses
- Functional constipation
    - Bulk forming laxatives (bran, ispaghula)
    - Bisacodyl or senna.
    - Lubiprostone
- Bedridden patients
    - For prevention—Bulk forming laxatives/docusates
    - For treatment—Bisacodyl/senna.

- To avoid straining—Hernia, cardiovascular disease, eye surgery, piles, anal surgery
  - Bulk forming/docusates.
- Preparation of bowel for surgery, colonoscopy, abdominal X-ray
  - Saline purgatives; alternatively bisacodyl (suppository).
- After niclosamide treatment
  - To wash of partially digested worm (*T. solium* → release of larvae → visceral cysticercosis)
  - Saline purgatives.
- Food/drug poisoning
  - Saline purgatives.

Diarrhea

An abnormal increase in frequency and liquidity of stools.
- Osmotic diarrhea—It is due to osmotic substances—Glycerine, lactose, magnesium-containing antacids
- Secretory diarrhea—Bacteria/virus/protozoa
- Motility disorder diarrhea—Irritable bowel syndrome (IBS), scleroderma, and diabetic neuropathy.

Pathophysiology

- Jejunum—Water and electrolytes are freely absorbed with nutrients.
- Ileum and colon—Na^+/K^+-ATPase mediated electrolyte absorption.

  Glucose facilitates Na^+ absorption in ileum and is intact even in severe diarrhea.

Management

Principle—Treat the fluid depletion and try to establish the underlying cause and give specific therapy if necessary.

Methods

- Fluid and electrolyte balance
  - Oral rehydration therapy (ORT)
  - Intravenous rehydration.
- Maintenance of nutrition.
- Drug therapy
  - Specific—Antimicrobials (ciprofloxacin, metronidazole, and diloxanide furoate).

- Nonspecific
  - Antisecretory drugs (sulfasalazine and mesalazine)
  - Antimotility drugs (codeine, diphenoxylate is combined with atropine and is available as Lomotil, and loperamide).

Fluid and Electrolyte Balance
Oral Rehydration Therapy (ORT)
5–7 mL/kg/h to 7.5–10 mL/kg/h (mild-to-moderate dehydration).
- Rationale of oral rehydration salt (ORS) solution
- Glucose—Facilitates Na^+ absorption from ileum
- It should be isotonic/hypotonic (200–310 mOsm/L)
- Molar ratio of glucose should be equal or slightly higher than Na^+
- Enough K^+ and bicarbonate/citrate → to replace the losses.

WHO—ORS Formula for Oral Rehydration Powder (One Sachet Contains)
- NaCl = 2.6 g
- KCl = 1.5 g
- Trisodium citrate = 2.9 g
- Glucose = 13.5 g
- To be dissolved in 1 liter of boiled and cooled water, this solution should be used within 24 hours
- With zinc supplement—10 mg/day (<6 months) and 20 mg/day (>6 months) for 10–14 days.

Advantages of Zinc Supplement
- ↓ the severity and duration of diarrhea; also prevents the diarrheal episode for 2–4 months.

Advantages of New ORS Formula
- More water absorption from hypotonic solution (due to ↓ Na and glucose)
- ↓ osmotic diarrhea (due to less glucose)
- Stool volume reduced by 20% and incidence of vomiting by 33%.

ANTIAMOEBIC AND ANTIPROTOZOAL DRUGS

Classifications
- Tissue amebicides
  - For intestinal and extraintestinal amebiasis—Metronidazole, tinidazole, secnidazole, satranidazole, emetine, dehydroemetine.
  - For extraintestinal only—Chloroquine.

- Luminal amebicides—Diloxanide furoate, quiniodochlor, tetracycline.

Treatment of Amebiasis
- Invasive intestinal amebiasis/amebic dysentery—Metronidazole/tinidazole (2 g single dose) followed by diloxanide furoate (500 mg tds for 5 days).
- Chronic intestinal amebiasis/asymptomatic cyst passers—Diloxanide furoate, metronidazole/tinidazole, tetracycline.
- Hepatic amebiasis—Metronidazole/tinidazole, dehydroemetine, diloxanide furoate, chloroquine.

Drugs for Giardiasis
- Metronidazole
- Mepacrine
- Quiniodochlor
- Furazolidone.

Drugs for Trichomoniasis
Orally
Metronidazole, nimorazole (2 g single dose with meal).

Intravaginally
- Diiodohydroxyquin
- Quiniodochlor
- Clotrimazole
- Natamycin.

ANTHELMINTICS
Nematodes—Thread like-spherical/cylindrical.

Classification Based on Location in the Body
- Intestinal nematodes
  - Small intestine—*Ascaris, Ancylostoma, Necator, Strongyloides,* and *Trichinella*
  - Large intestine—*Enterobius* and *Trichuris*.
- Tissue nematodes
  - Lymphatics—*Wuchereria, Brugia*
  - Subcutaneous—*Loa loa, Onchocerca,* and *Dracunculus*
  - Mesentery—*Mansonella*
  - Conjunctiva—*Loa loa*.

Classification Based on Mode of Infections
- By ingestion
  - Eggs—*Ascaris, Enterobius, Trichuris*
  - Larva—*Dracunculus*
  - Encysted larva in muscle—*Trichinella*.
- By penetration of skin—*Ancylostoma, Enterobius,* and *Trichuris*.
- By blood sucking insects—*Filariae*.
- By inhalation of dust containing eggs—*Ascaris* and *Enterobius*.

Cestodes—Ribbon/tape-like

Classification Based on Type of Sucker
- Pseudophyllidean (slit-like suckers) tapeworms
  - *Diphyllobothrium latum* (fish tapeworm)
- Cyclophyllidean tapeworms
  - *Taenia* → *T. saginata* (beef), *T. solium* (pork)
  - *Echinococcus* → *E. granulosus* (dog) and larval forms cause hydatid disease in human; *E. multilocularis*
  - *Hymenolepis* → *H. nana* (dwarf tapeworm).

Anthelmintics
- Mebendazole
- Albendazole
- Pyrantel pamoate
- Piperazine
- Levamisole, tetramisole
- Diethylcarbamazine citrate (DEC)
- Ivermectin
- Niclosamide
- Praziquantel.

Mebendazole
- Mechanism of action—Blocks glucose uptake and depletion of its glycogen stores → starvation → death
- Uses—Roundworm, hookworm, threadworm, and whipworm infestations
- Adverse drug reactions—GI upset, loss of hair, and granulocytopenia
  Albendazole—Similar to mebendazole.

Uses
- Ascaris, hookworm, whipworm, and enterobius infestation
- Tapeworm infestation and strongyloidiasis

- Neurocysticercosis
- Hydatid disease.

Pyrantel Pamoate
- Mechanism of action—It activates nicotic cholinergic receptors in the worm → persistent depolarization → contracture and spastic paralysis
- Adverse drug reaction—Very safe, sometimes GI upset, headache, and dizziness
- Uses—Infestation by *Ascaris, Ancylostoma, Enterobius, Necator,* and *Strongyloides.*

Piperazine
- Mechanism of action—Produces hyperpolarization of ascaris muscle by a gamma-amino butyric acid (GABA) receptor agonistic action opening Cl⁻ channels → flaccid paralysis
- Safe in pregnancy
- Uses—Infestation by *Ascaris* and *Enterobius.*

Levamisole, Tetramisole (Levoisomer of Levamisole)
- Mechanism of action—Stimulates the ganglia in worms → causes spastic/tonic paralysis; also inhibits fumarate reductase enzyme → interference with carbohydrate metabolism.
- Uses—Ascariasis and ancylostomiasis.

Diethylcarbamazine (DEC)
- Mechanism of action—It alters microfilariae (mf) membranes (*Wuchereria bancrofti* and *Brugia malayi*) → which are easily phagocytosed by tissue monocytes.
- Uses—Filariasis, tropical eosinophilia.
- Adverse drug reaction—Headache, nausea, loss of appetite; mass destructions of microfilariae and adult worms → fever, rash, pruritus, enlargement of lymph nodes.
- Treatment—Corticosteroids and antihistamines.

Ivermectin
- Mechanism of action—It acts through glutamate gated Cl⁻ channels → paralysis.
- Uses—Onchocerciasis, filariasis, orally (ivermectin is the only drug) in scabies and pediculosis.
- Adverse drug reaction—Pruritus, constipation, transient ECG changes, and reactions due to products of dead microfilariae.

Niclosamide

- Mechanism of action—It inhibits oxidative phosphorylation in mitochondria and interferes with ATP generation by the tapeworms.
- Uses—All types of tapeworm infestations [but not a first choice of drug, because of multiple doses, digestion of tapeworm (*Taenia solium*) → may release larva → visceral cysticercosis; so saline purgation is needed].
- Adverse drug reaction—Occasional GI upset.
- Safe in pregnancy.

Praziquantel

- Mechanism of action—It causes leakage of intracellular calcium → contracture and paralysis.
- Uses
  - Tapeworm infestations (all types)
  - Neurocysticercosis
  - Schistosomes.

First Choice of Drugs for Different Helminthic Infestations

Worm	Drug(s) of choice	Mechanism of action
Roundworm *Ascaris lumbricoides*	Albendazole, mebendazole, pyrantel, piperazine (in pregnancy)	*Albendazole, mebendazole:* ↓Microtubule assembly → blocks glucose uptake and depletion of its glycogen stores → starvation → death
		Pyrantel: Activates nicotinic cholinergic receptors in the worm → persistent depolarization → contracture and spastic paralysis of worms
		Piperazine: Activates GABA receptors → opening of Cl⁻ channels → hyperpolarization → flaccid paralysis of worms
Hookworm *Ancylostoma duodenale Necator americanus*	Albendazole, mebendazole, also pyrantel for Ancylostoma	See above

Contd...

Contd...

Worm	Drug(s) of choice	Mechanism of action
Pinworm *Enterobius (Oxyuris) vermicularis*	Albendazole, mebendazole, pyrantel	See above
Thread worm *Strongyloides stercoralis*	Ivermectin	*Ivermectin:* Activates glutamate gated Cl⁻ channels (found only in invertebrates), also activates GABA receptors→ ↑Cl⁻ influx into the cells→ paralysis of worms
Whipworm *Trichuris trichiura*	Mebendazole	See above
Trichinella spiralis	Albendazole	See above
Filaria *Wuchereria bancrofti, Brugia malayi*	Diethyl carbamazepine, Ivermectin	*Diethyl carbamazepine:* Alters microfilariae organelle membranes of *W. bancrofti* and *B. malayi* → which are easily phagocytosed by tissue monocytes *Ivermectin:* See above
Guineaworm *Dracunculus medinensis*	Metronidazole	*Metronidazole:* Anaerobic organisms/ameba/protozoa produce→ highly active nitro radicals from metronidazole by redox proteins (pyruvate: ferredoxin-oxidoreductase (PFOR))→ damage DNA→ cytotoxicity→ cell death
Tapeworms *Taenia saginata (beef)* *Taenia solium (pork)* *Hymenolepis nana (dwarf)*	Praziquantel	*Praziquantel:* Causes leakage of intracellular calcium → contracture and paralysis of worms
Neurocysticercosis	Albendazole	*Albendazole:* See above
Trematodes (flukes)	Praziquantel	*Praziquantel:* See above

COMMON ANTISPASMODICS

- Dicyclomine—Anticholinergic (Uses: Morning sickness, motion sickness, dysmenorrhea, irritable bowel syndrome [IBS])
- Hyoscyamine—Anticholinergic
- Oxybutynin—Anticholinergic (detrusor instability → frequency and urge incontinence)
- Flavoxate—Anticholinergic
- Drotaverine—Nonanticholinergic smooth muscle antispasmodic (intestinal, biliary, renal colic, IBS, uterine spasms)
- Alverine and peppermint oil.

IMPORTANT HEPATOTOXIC DRUGS

- Paracetamol, phenytoin—Hepatic cell injury
- Chlorpromazine, rifampicin, erythromycin, androgens—Cholestatic jaundice
- Isoniazid—Hepatitis
- Alcohol, methotrexate—Liver cirrhosis
- Halothane, enflurane—Immunologically-induced hepatitis.

CHAPTER 9

Autonomic Nervous System

CHOLINERGIC AND ANTICHOLINERGIC DRUGS

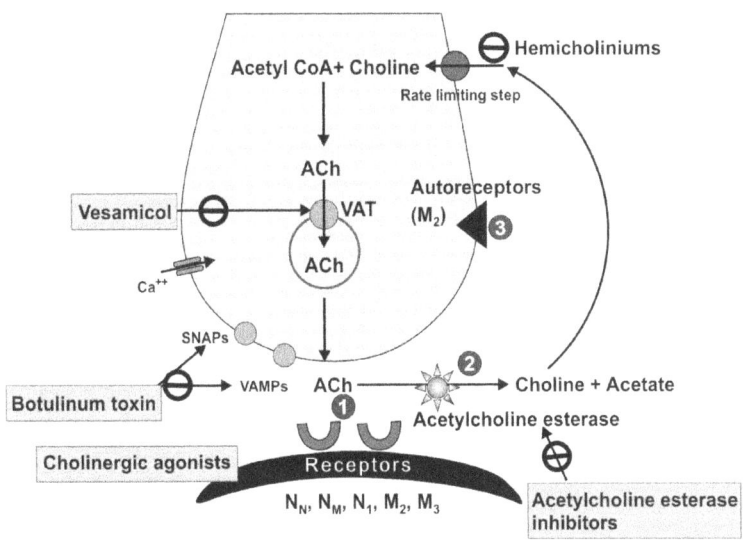

Cholinergic transmission and drugs acting (inhibitors and agonists) at different levels of synthesis, release, degradation, and receptors.

(VAT: vesicle-associated transporter, VAMPs: vesicle-associated membrane proteins, SNAPs: synaptosome-associated proteins, ACh: acetylcholine)

Numbers indicate major events after release of ACh. 1. Interaction of ACh with different cholinergic receptors (nicotinic and muscarinic at different tissues); 2. Degradation of ACh by acetylcholine esterase enzyme; 3. Auto-feedback inhibition of ACh release by ACh itself via M2 receptors

Classification of Cholinergic Receptors

Muscarinic: GPCRs → M_1 (neuronal), M_2 (cardiac), M_3 (smooth muscles); less understood—M_4, M_5.

Autonomic Nervous System

Table 9.1: Important locations and effects of cholinergic nicotinic receptors.

	N_N	N_M
Locations and effects	• Autonomic ganglia (PANS and SANS): Stimulation → depolarization → postganglionic impulse generation • Adrenal medulla → stimulation → release of epinephrine (mainly) and norepinephrine • CNS: Excitation or inhibition	Neuromuscular junction: Stimulation → depolarization → contraction of skeletal muscle
Nature	Ionotropic (ionic)	Ionotropic (ionic)
Transducer mechanisms	Opening of Na^+, K^+ channels	Opening of Na^+, K^+ channels

Table 9.2: Important locations and effects of cholinergic muscarinic receptors.

	M_1	M_2	M_3
Location and effects	• Neuronal: Autonomic ganglia (PANS and SANS) → stimulation → depolarization → postganglionic impulse generation • Gastric glands → histamine release → HCl secretion • CNS: Learning, memory, motor functions	• Cardiac: • SA node → hyperpolarization → bradycardia • AV node → hyperpolarization → ↓ conduction	• Smooth muscles: Iris: contraction → miosis • Ciliary muscle: contraction → spasm of accommodation • Vascular endothelium: release of NO (nitric oxide) → vasodilation
Nature	GPCR	GPCR (inhibitory)	GPCR
Transducer mechanisms	IP_3/DAG— ↑ cytosolic Ca^{++}	K^+ channel opening, ↓ cAMP	IP_3/DAG—↑ cytosolic Ca^{++}

(GPCR: G-protein coupled receptor; DAG: diacylglycerol; PANS: parasympathetic nervous system; SANS: sympathetic nervous system; IP3: inositol 1,4,5 triphosphate; NO: nitric oxide)

Note: M_2 is inhibitory.
Nicotinic: Ionic (ionotropic) → N_N (in ganglia), N_M (in neuromuscular junction)

Cholinergic Drugs
- Cholinesterase—Acetylcholine, methacholine
- Alkaloids—Muscarine, pilocarpine
- Anticholinesterase
  - Reversible—Physostigmine, neostigmine, edrophonium
  - Irreversible
    - Organophosphates—Dyflos, parathion, malathion
    - Carbamates—Carbaryl, propoxur.

Organophosphorus Poisoning
- Toxic features—30 min-3 h; most fatalities within 24 h and recovery within 10 days
- Muscarinic effects—Vomiting, diarrhea, abdominal cramps, bronchospasm, miosis, bradycardia, excessive salivation, and sweating
- Nicotinic effects—Muscle fasciculation, tremor and weakness; respiratory muscle paralysis, BP and pulse may ↑ or ↓
- CNS effects—Agitation, seizures, and comma.

Drugs Used in Organophosphorus Poisoning
Atropine (cholinergic muscarinic receptor antagonist, lipid-soluble crosses blood-brain barrier and antagonizes CNS muscarinic effects, drug of choice) and pralidoxime (it reactivates cholinesterase enzyme inhibited by the organophosphorus compounds if given within 2-3 h of poisoning).

Management of Organophosphorus Compound Poisoning
- Skin decontamination
- Gastric lavage (within 1 h of ingestion)
- Activated charcoal 0.5-1 g/kg every 4 h
- Anticholinergic: Atropine (drug of choice, lipid-soluble, antidote)
- Cholinesterase reactivator: Pralidoxime (contraindicated in carbamate poisoning)
- Ventilatory support to maintain proper oxygenation
- Inotropic support to ↑ the cardiac force of contraction →↑ cardiac output
- Feeding—Enteral/parenteral.

Uses of Cholinergic Drugs
- As miotics
  - In glaucoma (physostigmine)
  - To counteract the effect of mydriatics after refraction testing
  - To prevent formation of adhesions between lens or iris and cornea
- Myasthenia gravis (neostigmine)
- Postoperative paralytic ileus/urinary retention (neostigmine)
- Postoperative decurarization (neostigmine)
- Cobra bite–Cobra venom has curare like neurotoxin (neostigmine + atropine)
- Belladonna (atropine) poisoning (physostigmine)
- Alzheimer's disease (rivastigmine, donepezil).

Side Effects of Cholinergic Drugs
- Lacrimation
- Sialorrhea
- Increased sweating
- Bronchospasm
- Peptic ulcer
- Abdominal cramps
- Diarrhea
- Miosis
- Eyes become fixed to near vision
- Spasm of accommodation (due to contraction of ciliary muscle).

Anticholinergic Drugs
- Natural alkaloids—Atropine, hyoscine
- Semisynthetic—Homatropine, ipratropium bromide, tiotropium bromide
- Synthetic—Tropicamide (mydriatic), glycopyrrolate (antisecretory), dicyclomine (antispasmodic), trihexyphenidyl (antiparkinsonian).

Uses of Anticholinergic (Antimuscarinic Drugs)
- As antisecretory
  - Preanesthetic medication (glycopyrrolate— ↓ salivary and tracheobronchial secretions → prevent reflex laryngospasm).
  - Peptic ulcer (propantheline, oxyphenonium)
  - Hyperhidrosis (darifenacin), excessive salivation (dicyclomine).

- As antispasmodic
  - Intestinal and renal colic (atropine methonitrate, dicyclomine)
  - Nervous and drug induced diarrhea, functional diarrhea (atropine, oxyphenonium)
  - Urinary urge incontinence, enuresis (oxybutynin, flavoxate).
- COPD and bronchial asthma
  - Ipratropium bromide and tiotropium bromide (COPD—As prophylaxis; bronchial asthma with β_2-agonist in acute exacerbation).
- As mydriatic and cycloplegic
  - To test error of refraction-tropicamide (quickest and briefest)—Both mydriasis and cycloplegia.
  - Fundoscopy—Only mydriasis is required—Phenylephrine (no ocular side effects and fear of precipitation of glaucoma).
  - Treatment of iridocyclitis/iritis/uveitis—Homatropine → provides rest to intraocular muscles, prevents painful spasms, and when used with pilocarpine alternately, prevents adhesions between iris and anterior surface of the lens.
- As cardiac vagolytic: Bradycardia and partial heart block—Atropine, tripitamine (M2 selective blocker)
- Prophylaxis for motion sickness: Hyoscine (transdermal patch, placed behind the pinna 4 h before journey—3 days)
- Parkinsonism (drug-induced): Trihexyphenidyl (benzhexol), biperiden
- To antagonize muscarinic effects of drugs and poisons
- Anticholinesterase (organophosphorus) and early type of mushroom poisoning—Atropine
- Neostigmine therapy in myasthenia gravis—Atropine to block muscarinic actions
- Decurarization and cobra envenomation—Neostigmine + atropine.

Side Effects of Anticholinergic Drugs
- Dry or sandy eyes (due to ↓ lacrimation)
- Xerostomia (dry mouth, due to ↓ salivation)
- Dry skin (due to ↓ sweating)
- Constipation
- Urinary retention
- Photophobia
- Mydriasis
- Eyes become fixed to the distant vision (due to cycloplegia).

ADRENERGIC DRUGS AND ANTIADRENERGIC DRUGS

Classification of Adrenergic Receptors
- Alpha receptors: GPCRs → α_1 (postsynaptic, excitatory), α_2 (presynaptic, inhibitory)
- Beta receptors: GPCRs → β_1 (cardiac), β_2 (airway tract and lungs), β_3 (fat cells, stimulation → ↑ lipolysis).

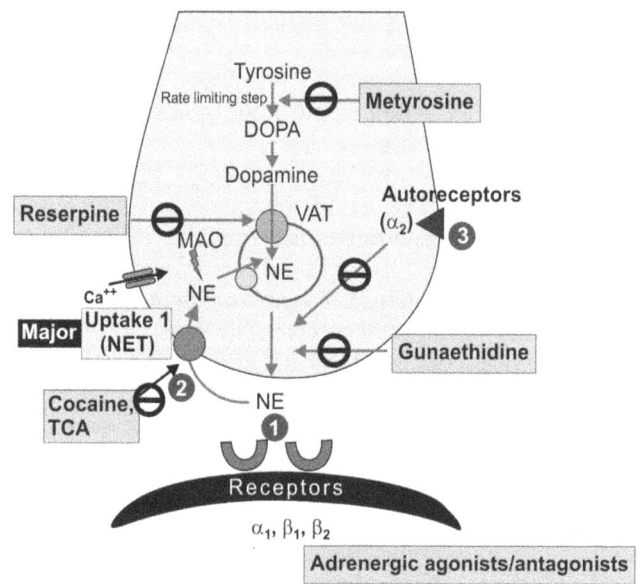

Adrenergic transmission and drugs acting (inhibitors and agonists) at different levels of synthesis, release, uptake, and receptors.

(TCA: tricyclic antidepressant; NET: norepinephrine transporter, VAT: vesicle associated transporter; MAO: monoamine oxidase; DOPA: dihydroxyphenylalanine)

Numbers indicate major events after release of NE. 1. Interaction of NE with different adrenergic receptors; 2. Neuronal re-uptake of NE; 3. Feedback inhibition of NE by NE itself via alpha-2 receptors

Adrenergic Drugs
- Catecholamines—Adrenaline, noradrenaline, and dopamine
- Noncatecholamine—Ephedrine and amphetamine.

Therapeutic Classifications
- Pressure agents—Noradrenaline, ephedrine, and dopamine
- Cardiac stimulants—Adrenaline, isoprenaline, and dobutamine

Table 9.3: Important locations and effects of adrenergic receptors.

	α₁	α₂
Locations and effects	• Peripheral blood vessels: Vasoconstriction → ↑ total peripheral resistance →↑ BP • Dilator pupillae: Mydriasis (pupillary dilation) • Bladder trigone: Contraction (urinary retention) • Arrector pilorum: Piloerection (goose bumps)	• Presynaptic neuronal membrane: ↓ release of the neurotransmitter (mostly NE) → ↓ sympathetic outflow (↓ BP, ↓ HR) • Pancreatic beta cells: ↓ insulin release
Nature	GPCR	GPCR (inhibitory)
Transducer mechanisms	IP₃/DAG—↑ cytosolic Ca⁺⁺	↓ cAMP

	β₁	β₂
Locations and effects	• Heart (SA and AV node, muscle fibers): Cardiac stimulation (positive chronotropic, dromotropic and inotropic effects →↑ HR, CO) • Kidney (juxta-glomerular cells): ↑ Renin secretion → ↑ renin–angiotensin–aldosterone system →↑ BP	Smooth muscles: • Bronchus: Bronchodilation • Arterioles: Vasodilatation (coronary, skeletal muscles) • Uterus: Relaxation → delays labor Liver cells: Glycogenolysis →↑ in blood glucose Skeletal muscle: Muscle tremor (hand tremor)
Nature	GPCR	GPCR
Transducer mechanisms	↑ cAMP	↑ cAMP

- Bronchodilators—Salbutamol and salmeterol
- CNS stimulants—Amphetamine and methamphetamine.

Uses

- Vascular uses
    - Hypotensive states
    - Along with local anesthetics

- Control of local bleeding
- Nasal decongestant
- Peripheral vascular diseases.
* Cardiac uses
  - Cardiac arrest
  - Partial or complete A-V block
  - Congestive heart failure.
* Bronchial asthma
* As mydriatic
* Central uses
  - Narcolepsy
  - Attention deficit hyperkinetic disorder
  - Obesity.
* Nocturnal enuresis in children and urinary incontinence
* Uterine relaxant.

Side Effects of Adrenergic Medicines
* Increase blood pressure
* Palpitation
* Anxiety
* Insomnia
* Nightmare
* Aggression
* Hyperglycemia
* Anorexia.

Antiadrenergic Drugs
* α-blockers—Phenoxybenzamine, phentolamine, prazosin, terazosin, yohimbine
* β-blockers—Propranolol, timolol, pindolol, labetalol, carvedilol, atenolol, metoprolol.

Uses of α-blockers
* Pheochromocytoma
* Hypertension with benign prostatic hypertension (BPH)
* BPH.

Side Effects of α-blockers
* Postural hypotension
* Palpitation
* Dizziness.

Uses of β-blockers
- Hypertension
- Cardiac arrhythmia
- Congestive cardiac failure (only in stable patients)
- Angina pectoris (stable angina)
- Hyperthyroidism.

Side Effects of β-blockers
- Bradycardia
- Bronchoconstriction
- Glucose intolerance
- Rebound hypertension (if withdrawn suddenly).

MYDRIATICS AND MIOTICS

Mydriasis—Pupillary Dilatation
Fright, sudden emotional state, first and third stage of anesthesia, hysteria, drugs (atropine, cocaine, ephedrine, homatropine) cause mydriasis.

Mydriatic—Drug that Causes Pupillary Dilatation
Mydriatics
- Anticholinergics (antimuscarinic)—Atropine, homatropine, cyclopentolate, tropicamide, scopolamine.
- Adrenergic—Phenylephrine.

Uses of Mydriatics
- Diagnostic to test error of refraction (both mydriasis and cycloplegia are needed); for fundoscopy (only mydriasis is required) → tropicamide or phenylephrine.
- Therapeutic to prevent the adhesions in inflammatory conditions → atropine or homatropine is alternated with miotics (e.g. pilocarpine) to prevent the adhesion between iris and anterior surface of the lens in iridocyclitis, iritis, and uveitis.

Atropine—ADR-eyes become fixed to distant vision, dry (red) eyes, burning sensation in the eyes.

Miosis (Gr—Meiosis)—A Lessening
Typhus fever, early stages of meningitis, opioid poisoning (morphine and similar drugs), pontine hemorrhage, sunstroke, cholinergic drugs → cause miosis.

Miotic—Drug that Causes Pupillary Constriction
Commonly used miotics
- Pilocarpine 0.5%
- Physostigmine 0.1%.
  Others (not used)—Echothiophate, isoflurophate (more side effects).

Uses
- In glaucoma (open angle, wide angle, chronic).
- With mydriatics alternatively to break adhesions during ocular inflammatory conditions.

LOCAL ANESTHETIC AGENTS
Classifications
- On the basis of chemical structure
  - Esters
    Cocaine, benzocaine, procaine, tetracaine
  - Amides
    Bupivacaine, etidocaine, lidocaine, mepivacaine, prilocaine.
- On the basis of duration of action
  - Ultrashort-acting (<30 min)
    2% lignocaine without vasoconstrictor
  - Short-acting (<90 min)
    2% lignocaine with vasoconstrictor
  - Medium-acting (90–150 min)
    4% prilocaine with vasoconstrictor
  - Long-acting (≥180 min)
    0.5% bupivacaine with vasoconstrictor 1.5% etidocaine with vasoconstrictor
    (Vasoconstrictor—Adrenaline—1:80,000).

Mechanism of Actions
- Block Na^+ channels (from inside; resting channels-resistant) → prevent the development of AP → no stimulation of nerve fiber → stop conduction
- Local anesthesia → Block every type of nerve fiber
- Channel recovery rate—10–1,000 times slower.

Local Anesthesia with Vasoconstrictor
Advantages
- ↑ Duration of action
- ↓ Systemic toxicity
- Relatively more bloodless surgery.

Disadvantages
- It may cause necrosis
- ↓ Wound healing
- It may increase BP, tachycardia.

Effects of Local Anesthesia
- Local—Nerves at the site of injection.
- Systemic.
- *Local effects:*
  - Differential nerve block
    - Smaller fibers, nonmyelinated, high frequency, autonomic fibers → more sensitive.
    - Somatic afferents—pain → temperature → touch → pressure.
- *Systemic effects:*
  - Central nervous system
    - Inhibit inhibitory neurons—Convulsion
    - Stimulation followed by depression (cocaine is powerful stimulant).
  - Central venous system
    - Cardiac depression (antiarrhythmic drugs)
    - Vasodilatation →↓ BP (except-cocaine →↑ BP and HR).
- *Blood*
- Prilocaine→metabolite (o-toluidine) → methemoglobinemia → Cyanosis
- Lidocaine/lignocaine
  - Synthesized in 1943 by Lofgren
  - Most widely used local anesthesia
  - Good for surface application as well as injection
  - Blocks conduction within 3 min
  - It is used for surface application, infiltration, nerve block, epidural, spinal, and IV regional block anesthesia
  - Central effects—Drowsiness, mental clouding
  - Overdose—Muscle twitching, convulsions, cardiac arrhythmias, fall in BP, coma, and respiratory arrest
  - Popular antiarrhythmic (blocks cardiac Na^+ channels in ventricular and atrial muscles).
- Bupivacaine
  - Potent and long-lasting amide
  - It is used for infiltration, nerve block, and epidural and spinal anesthesia of long duration

- A 0.25-0.5% solution injected epidurally produces adequate analgesia without significant motor blockade
- Very popular in obstetrics and for postoperative pain relief
- High lipid solubility
- It is distributed more in tissues than in blood after, spinal/epidural injection—Less likely to reach the fetus
- More prone to induce ventricular tachycardia and cardiac depression (death reports—at 0.75% bupivacaine)
- It should not be used for IV regional analgesia.

CHAPTER 10

Central Nervous System

GENERAL ANESTHETIC AGENTS

Produce reversible loss of all sensation (especially pain) and consciousness.

Cardinal Features
- Loss of all sensation
- Unconsciousness and amnesia
- Immobility
- Abolition of reflexes.

Minimum Alveolar Concentration (MAC)
- Lowest concentration of anesthetic in pulmonary alveoli needed to produce immobility in response to a painful stimuli in 50% individuals.
- Measure of potency.

Mechanism of Anesthesia
Exact mechanism—Not known.
- However, they cause degree of disorder in the cell membrane—affect the state of membrane bound functional proteins and/or expand the membrane disproportionately (approximately 10 times) → closure of ion channels.

  This generalized hypothesis has been replaced by agent specific theories. Agent specific theory states that different agents produce anesthesia by different mechanisms. The following are the well-understood mechanisms:
- Many inhalational anesthetics, barbiturates, benzodiazepines, and propofol → potentiate the action of gamma-aminobutyric acid (GABA) at $GABA_A$ →↑ Cl^- entry.
- Ketamine and N_2O—inhibit the N-methyl-D-aspartate (NMDA) type of glutamate receptor →↓ Ca^{++} entry.

- Some fluorinated anesthetics and barbiturates → also inhibit the neuronal cation channel gated by cholinergic receptor.
  Local anesthesias—block axonal conduction.
  General anesthesias—Depress synaptic transmission.

Techniques of Inhalation of Anesthetics
- Open drop method
- Through anesthetic machines
  - *Open system*—Rebreathing in the anesthetic machine is not allowed, used for nonexpensive anesthetic agents.
  - *Closed system*—Rebreathing is allowed, used for expensive anesthetic agents, exhaled mixture passes through soda lime to absorb CO_2.
  - *Semiclosed system*—Partial rebreathing is allowed.

Classifications
- Inhalational
  - Gas—Nitrous oxide
  - Liquid—Ether, halothane, enflurane, isoflurane, sevoflurane, desflurane.
- Intravenous
  - Inducing agents: Thiopentone sodium, propofol, etomidate.
  - Slower acting agents
    - Benzodiazepines—Diazepam, lorazepam, midazolam
    - Dissociative anesthesia—Ketamine
    - Opioid analgesia—Fentanyl.

Complications of General Anesthesia that may arise during and after
- Malignant hyperthermia (with halothane, succinylcholine)
- Respiratory depression
- Emergence reactions—Disorientation, excitation, and hallucinations (ketamine)
- Salivation, ↑ respiratory secretion
- Cardiac arrhythmias (fluorinated anesthetic agents)
- ↓ Blood pressure (BP)
- Laryngospasm and asphyxia
- Nausea, vomiting
- Aspiration pneumonia.

SEDATIVES AND HYPNOTICS
Sedative Agent
It should reduce anxiety and exert a calming effect.

Hypnotic Agent
It should produce drowsiness and encourage the onset and maintenance of sleep.

Classifications
- Barbiturates:
    - Long-acting—Phenobarbitone and mephobarbital
    - Short-acting—Pentobarbital, secobarbital, and amobarbital
    - Ultrashort-acting—Thiopentone and methohexital.

    As sedative/hypnotic (because they are more toxic, have low therapeutic index than benzodiazepines), they are obsolete and only used in anesthesia (thiopentone) and in epilepsy (generalized tonic-clonic seizure—Phenobarbitone).
- Benzodiazepines
    - Hypnotic—Diazepam, flurazepam, and midazolam
    - Sedative/antianxiety—Diazepam, chlordiazepoxide, oxazepam, lorazepam, and alprazolam
    - Anticonvulsant—Diazepam, lorazepam, clobazam, clonazepam, nitrazepam, and clorazepate
    - Based on duration of action
        - Long-acting (t½ 30-100 hours)—Flurazepam, diazepam, and nitrazepam
        - Short-acting (t½ 2-12 hours)—Alprazolam, temazepam, and triazolam
- Newer nonbenzodiazepine agents—Zolpidem, zopiclone, and zaleplon
- Miscellaneous
    - Partial agonist at $5HT_{1A}$ receptor—Buspirone
    - Melatonin receptor agonist—Ramelteon
    - Antihistaminics—Promethazine, diphenhydramine, and hydroxyzine
    - Older agents—Chloral hydrate, paraldehyde, and meprobamate.

Barbiturates and benzodiazepines act through $GABA_A$ receptor which is ionotropic receptor → after binding with the receptor → influx of Cl⁻ ions (barbiturates increase the *duration of chloride channel opening* whereas benzodiazepines increase the *frequency of chloride channel opening*) → hyperpolarization (remember that inside of the cell is negative potential) → depression of the electrical activity which is required for the generation of action potential.

Flumazenil is benzodiazepine antagonist and can be used in case of benzodiazepine overdose.

Uses of Benzodiazepines
- Treatment of anxiety states
- Treatment of sleep disorders (insomnia)
- Seizures—Control of status epilepticus, febrile convulsions, tetanus
- As centrally acting muscle relaxant
- Preanesthetic medication
- Alcohol withdrawal in dependent subjects
- In psychiatry-electroconvulsive therapy
- Others—Electrical cardioversion of arrhythmias, cardiac catheterization, endoscopies.

Side Effects of Benzodiazepines
- Daytime sedation, drowsiness
- Vertigo, ataxia
- Hangover—Drowsiness, dysphoria, mental and motor depression the following day
- Aggravate obstructive sleep apnea
- Psychomotor impairment, impaired judgment and cognitive function, anterograde amnesia
- Tolerance, psychological and physiological dependence
- Synergistic depression of central nervous system (CNS) with other CNS depressants.

ANXIOLYTIC AGENTS

Classifications
- Benzodiazepine (BZD): Diazepam, chlordiazepoxide, oxazepam, lorazepam, alprazolam.
- Azapirone: Buspirone.
- Sedative antihistaminic: Hydroxyzine.
- β-blocker—Propranolol: In performance anxiety in which there is sympathetic overactivity.

ANTIDEPRESSANTS AND MOOD STABILIZERS

Antidepressants
- Drugs which elevate mood in depressive illness mostly affect monoaminergic transmission in the brain

Central Nervous System

- Effect on reuptake/metabolism of biogenic amines and on pre/postjunctional aminergic/cholinergic receptors.

Classifications
- Reversible inhibitors of monoamine oxidase-A (MAO-A)—Moclobemide, clorgyline
- Tricyclic antidepressants (TCAs)
  - Noradrenaline (NA) + 5-HT reuptake inhibitors—Imipramine, amitriptyline
  - Predominantly NA reuptake inhibitors—Desipramine, nortriptyline
- Selective serotonin reuptake inhibitors (SSRIs)—Fluoxetine, sertraline
- Atypical antidepressants—Trazodone, venlafaxine.

Uses of Antidepressants
- Endogenous (major) depression—SSRIs, TCA, Li
- Obsessive—Compulsive and phobic states—SSRIs, clomipramine (TCA)
- Anxiety disorders—BZD, SSRIs
- Neuropathic pain—Imipramine
- Attention deficit—Hyperactive disorder in children—Amphetamine, imipramine, nortriptyline
- Enuresis—Imipramine
- Migraine—Amitriptyline (prophylaxis).

Mood Stabilizers/Antimanic Drugs
- Lithium carbonate
- Alternative to lithium—Carbamazepine, sodium valproate, lamotrigine, olanzapine.

Mechanism of Actions
- Inhibits hydrolysis of inositol-1-phosphate → decrease in the regeneration of phosphatidylinositol biphosphate
- Decreases NA and dopamine release from the nerve terminals
- Plasma concentration
  - 0.8–1.1 mEq/L—Acute mania
  - 0.5–0.8 mEq/L—Maintenance therapy.

ANTIPSYCHOTICS
- Antipsychotics/neuroleptics—Major tranquilizers
- Anxiolytics/sedatives—Minor tranquilizers.

Psychiatric Disorders

- Psychoses
  - Organic psychosis (due to organic disease—cerebral infection by rabies or brain injuries, chronic alcoholism). Acute and chronic organic brain syndromes (cognitive disorders)—Dementia, disorientation, and disorganized behavior.
  - Functional psychosis (due to biochemical alteration in neurotransmitter levels in the brain):
    - Schizophrenia (introvert, no coherence between their thought, speech, and action)—Illusions, hallucinations, memory is usually retained.
    - Paranoid state/schizophrenia—Delusions are paranoid and persecutory in nature.
- Affective disorders (disorders of mood):
  - Mania
  - Depression
  - Bipolar disorder.
- Neuroses (less severe, personality is intact, no loss of contact with reality):
  - Anxiety
  - Phobic states
  - Obsessive compulsive disorder
  - Reactive depression
  - Post-traumatic stress disorder.

Psychotics make castle in the air and live there and neurotics make the castle in the air but they do not live there. Psychiatrists are so smart that they collect rent from the both (with due respect to psychiatrists). (*Source*: Principles of Pharmacology, by KK Sharma and HL Sharma).

Pathophysiology
- Dopamine (DA) hypothesis— ↑ DA activity
- 5-HT hypothesis—LSD, 5-HT_2 receptor agonist → hallucinations, similar to psychosis
- Glutamate hypothesis— ↓ NMDA receptor activity (no drug is available based on this hypothesis so far).

Classifications
- Phenothiazines—Chlorpromazine, prochlorperazine
- Butyrophenones—Haloperidol
- Thioxanthenes—Thiothixene
- Atypical neuroleptics—Clozapine, risperidone, olanzapine.

Uses
- *Psychiatric uses*
  - Schizophrenia
  - Mania
  - Organic brain syndrome.
- *Nonpsychiatric uses*
  - As antiemetics—Prochlorperazine
  - Preanesthetic medication—Chlorpromazine
  - Intractable hiccups—Chlorpromazine.

ANTIEPILEPTICS

Epilepsy
- Seizure—Paroxysmal abnormal discharge at high frequency from an aggregate of neurons in cerebral cortex.
- Epilepsy—Recurrent episodes of such seizures with or without loss of consciousness.
- Convulsions—Involuntary, violent, and spasmodic or prolonged contraction of skeletal muscle.
- Fit—Colloquial term for an epileptic seizure
- 1% of world population—These have been affected by epilepsy.

Classification of Seizures
- *Generalized*
  - Tonic-clonic or grand mal
    Repeated grand mal seizures without recovery in-between attacks → status epilepticus
  - Absence or petit mal (minor epilepsy)
  - Atonic seizure (akinetic epilepsy)
  - Myoclonic
  - Clonic seizure.
- *Partial seizures*
  - Simple partial seizures (cortical focal epilepsy)
  - Complex partial seizures (temporal lobe epilepsy/psychomotor epilepsy)
  - Partial seizure evolving to secondary generalized seizures.
- *Unclassified seizures*
  - Febrile seizures
  - Infantile spasm.

Pathogenesis

Most of the cases are primary (idiopathic) and some may be secondary:
- Increased firing of neurons due to Na^+ channels
- Decreased inhibition, i.e., ↓ GABA
- Increased concentration of excitatory amino acids glutamate, aspartate
- Increased entry of T-type Ca^{++} currents.

Classification of Drugs
- Prolongation of Na^+ channel inactivation—Phenytoin, carbamazepine, valproate, lamotrigine, zonisamide
- Facilitation of GABA mediated Cl^- channel opening —Barbiturate, benzodiazepine, vigabatrin, valproate, gabapentin, tiagabine, progabide
- Inhibition of T type Ca^{++} current—Ethosuximide, trimethadione, valproate, zonisamide
- Blockade of NMDA receptor—Felbamate.

Newer Antiepileptic Drugs
- Gabapentin, topiramate, lamotrigine
- Tiagabine, vigabatrin, levetiracetam
- Ganaxolone, progabide, zonisamide
- Felbamate

$MgSO_4^-$ drug of choice in preeclampsia and eclampsia of pregnancy.

OPIOID ANALGESICS

- Pain—Unpleasant sensation which usually arises from noxious stimuli
- Analgesic agent—Relieves pain
- *Types:*
  - Opioid/morphine like/centrally acting
  - Nonopioid/aspirin like/peripherally acting.

Classifications
- Natural opium alkaloids morphine, methylmorphine (codeine)
- Semisynthetic opiates diacetylmorphine (heroin)
- Synthetic opioids pethidine, fentanyl, methadone tramadol, dextropropoxyphene.

Morphine
- Named after Greek God of dreams "Morpheus"
- Principle alkaloid in opium
- Brown, resinous, material obtained from poppy (*Papaver somniferum*) capsule → opium.

Actions of Morphine

CNS

Depressant's actions
- Analgesic action—Strong analgesic.
  - Spinal action—It acts in the substantia gelatinosa of dorsal horn to inhibit release of excitatory transmitters; decrease release of substance P from primary pain afferents in the spinal cord.
  - Supraspinal action—It acts in medulla, midbrain, limbic cortical areas → alters processing and interpretation of pain impulses; also sends inhibitory impulses to the spinal cord.
- Sedation—Drowsiness and indifference to surrounding as well as own body.
- Mood and subjective effects
  - Calming effect, loss of apprehension
  - Inability to concentrate
  - Rapid IV injection—Causes "kick" or "rush," intensely pleasurable and akin to orgasm
  - Euphoria.
- Respiratory center
  - Depressed (both rate and tidal volume ↓)
  - In poisoning → respiratory failure → death.
- Cough center—Depressed more sensitive than respiratory center.
- Temperature regulation center—Hypothermia.
- Vasomotor center—Fall in BP (at higher doses).

Stimulatory Effects
- Chemoreceptor trigger zone (CTZ)
- Edinger-Westphal nucleus → stimulation → miosis → pin-point pupil (characteristic in opioid addicts)
- Vagal center
- Certain cortical areas and hippocampal cells:
  - Muscular rigidity and immobility
  - Convulsions (↓ GABA release).

Neuroendocrine
- Follicle-stimulating hormone (FSH), luteinizing hormone (LH), adrenocorticotropic hormone (ACTH), antidiuretic hormone (ADH) ↓
- Prolactin and growth hormone ↑
- Infertility may occur in addicts.

CVS
- Vasodilation
- ↓ Tone of blood vessels
- Histamine release
- Depression of vasomotor center
- ↓ Preload, ↓ afterload.

GIT
- Constipation (↓ propulsive movements)
- No tolerance develops to this action → addicts remain chronically constipated.

Other smooth muscles
- Biliary tract—Spasm of sphincter of Oddi →↑ intrabiliary pressure ↑ biliary colic
- Urinary bladder—↑ the tone of detrusor and sphincter ↑ difficulty in micturation
- Bronchi—Bronchoconstriction (due to ↑ histamine release).

Adverse Drug Reactions
- Sedation, vomiting, mental clouding, lethargy
- Idiosyncrasy and allergy
- Apnea
- Respiratory depression
- Blurring of vision
- Urinary retention
- Tolerance (except miosis and constipation)
- Dependence (both psychological and physical)
- Abuse liability.

Morphine Withdrawal Syndrome
- Lacrimation, sweating, restlessness, fear
- Anxiety, mydriasis, tremor, insomnia
- Diarrhea, dehydration
- ↑ BP, palpitation.

Treatment
Withdrawal of morphine and substitution with oral methadone (long-acting, orally effective) followed by gradual withdrawal of methadone.

Acute Morphine Poisoning
Treatment
- Respiratory support
- Maintenance of BP (IV fluids and vasoconstrictors)
- Gastric lavage
- Naloxone (specific antidote).

Precautions and Contraindications
- Infants (apnea), elderly (urinary retention)
- Patients with respiratory insufficiency (emphysema, pulmonary fibrosis, cor pulmonale)
- Bronchial asthma (histamine release)
- Head injury (↑CO_2 retention, vomiting, miosis, altered sensorium)
- Hypotensive states
- Undiagnosed acute abdominal pain
- Unstable personalities (liable to continue).

Opioid Receptors
- μ-receptors—Morphine (high affinity)
- δ-receptors
- κ-receptors.

Complex Opioid Agonist-antagonist
- Agonist-antagonist
  - Pentazocine—It is used as analgesic.
- Pure antagonist
  - Naloxone, naltrexone.
- Endogenous opioid peptides
  - Endorphins
  - Enkephalins
  - Dynorphins.

Uses of Morphine and its Congeners
- As analgesic—Severe pain of any type:
  - Traumatic pain
  - Cancer pain
  - Myocardial infarction

- Burn
- Postoperative pain.
- Preanesthetic medication
  - Morphine/pethidine IM
  - Decrease fear and anxiety.
- Surgical anesthesia—Fentanyl IV
- Acute left ventricular failure
- Dry cough—Codeine
- Diarrhea—Codeine.

Alternate Routes of Opioid Administration
- Rectal suppositories—Morphine and hydromorphine
- Transdermal patch—Fentanyl
- Intranasal—Butorphanol
- Buccal—Fentanyl citrate lozenge or a lollipop
- Patient controlled analgesia (PCA)—Patient controls a parenteral (usually IV) infusion device by depressing a programmed dose of the desired opioid analgesic.

CHAPTER 11

Integumentary System

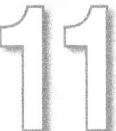

ANTIFUNGAL DRUGS

Classifications
- Antibiotics—Amphotericin B (AMB), nystatin, griseofulvin
- Antimetabolites—Flucytosine
- Azoles
  - *Topical*—Clotrimazole, econazole, miconazole, ketoconazole (KTZ)
  - *Systemic*—KTZ, fluconazole, itraconazole
- Others—Terbinafine, benzoic acid.

Amphotericin B

Mechanism of Actions
- It combines with ergosterol present in the fungal cell membrane, gets inserted into the membrane, and forms micropore →↑ membrane permeability.
- Fungicidal at high concentration and fungistatic at low concentration.

Uses
- Oral, vaginal, and cutaneous candidiasis
- Otomycosis
- Various types of systemic mycosis
- Leishmaniasis—Resistant cases of kala-azar and mucocutaneous leishmaniasis.

Adverse Effects

High Toxicity
- Acute reactions
  - Chills, fever, nausea, vomiting, dyspnea (due to release of IL, TNFα).
  - Thrombophlebitis of injected vein.

- Chronic toxicity
  - Nephrotoxicity
  - Anemia (due to bone marrow depression)
  - CNS toxicity—Headache, nerve palsies.

Liposomal amphotericin B preparation—Less adverse drug reactions.

Nystatin
- Similar to AMB
- It has higher systemic toxicity, so used only locally.

Griseofulvin
- Fungistatic
- Interferes with mitosis → multinucleated fungal hyphae
- It gets deposited in keratin forming cells of skin, hair, and nail
- Toxicity is low (headache and GI disturbances)
- It is used systemically only for dermatophytosis
- It is ineffective topically.

Flucytosine
- Inhibitor of thymidylate synthesis
- It is used as an adjuvant drug.

Azoles
- Clotrimazole, econazole, miconazole, KTZ—Topical
- KTZ, fluconazole, itraconazole—Systemically used.

Mechanism of Actions
- Inhibit the fungal cytochrome P_{450} lanosterol 14-demethylase → impair ergosterol synthesis → membrane abnormalities in fungus.
- Primarily fungistatic.

Clotrimazole

Uses
- Tinea infections
- Oral, cutaneous, and vaginal candidiasis
- Otomycosis.

Adverse Drug Reactions
- Local irritation (stinging and burning sensation)
- No systemic toxicity after topical use.

Econazole
- Similar to clotrimazole
- But inferior to clotrimazole in vaginal candidiasis.

Miconazole
- Highly efficacious
- Higher vaginal irritation than with clotrimazole.

Ketoconazole (KTZ)
- First orally effective broad spectrum antifungal
- Effective in both dermatophytosis and deep mycoses.

Adverse Drug Reactions
- Nausea, vomiting
- Loss of appetite, headache
- ↓ Androgen production in males → gynecomastia, loss of hair, loss of libido, oligozoospermia
- Menstrual irregularities in females.

Uses
- Dermatophytosis
- Vaginal candidiasis
- Systemic mycosis.

Contraindications
- Pregnancy
- Nursing women.

Fluconazole
Wider range of activity than KTZ.

Uses
- Cryptococcal meningitis
- Systemic and mucosal candidiasis
- Histoplasmosis.

Adverse Drug Reactions
- Less side effects than with KTZ (no antiandrogenic effects)
- Nausea, vomiting, headache.

Itraconazole
- Newer orally active antifungal
- Broader spectrum of activity than KTZ and fluconazole.

Uses
- Preferred to KTZ for many systemic mycosis
- Systemic mycosis
- Vaginal candidiasis
- Dermatophytosis
- Onychomycosis.

Integumentary System

Adverse Drug Reactions
- Gastric intolerance
- Dizziness, headache, hypokalemia, pruritus.

Terbinafine

Orally and topically active against dermatophytosis and *Candida*.

Mechanism of Actions
- It is fungicidal.
- Competitive inhibitor of squalene epoxidase (an initial enzyme in ergosterol synthesis) → accumulation of squalene within fungal cells.

Uses
- Tinea infections
- Pityriasis versicolor
- Onychomycosis.

Adverse Drug Reactions
- Erythema, itching, rashes
- Gastric upset, taste disturbance
- Hepatic dysfunction.

ANTIVIRAL DRUGS

Classifications
- Antiherpes virus: Idoxuridine, acyclovir, ganciclovir, and foscarnet.
- Antiretrovirus:
  - Nucleoside reverse transcriptase inhibitors (NRTIs): Zidovudine (AZT), didanosine, zalcitabine, stavudine, and lamivudine.
  - Nonnucleoside reverse transcriptase inhibitors (NNRTIs): Nevirapine, delavirdine, and efavirenz
  - Protease inhibitors: Ritonavir, indinavir, and saquinavir.
- Anti-influenza virus: Amantadine and rimantadine.

Antiherpes Virus

Idoxuridine

Mechanism of Action

It is pyrimidine antimetabolite and acts as a thymidine analog → faulty DNA synthesis → synthesis of wrong viral proteins → noninfective virus.

Uses
Herpes simplex and keratoconjunctivitis.

Side Effects
- Ocular irritation
- Edema of lids
- Photophobia.

Acyclovir
Mechanism of Action
Acyclovir is acted upon by virus specific thymidine kinase → acyclovir monophosphate is acted upon by cellular kinase → acyclovir triphosphate →↓ viral DNA synthesis.

Herpes simplex type I > herpes simplex type II > varicella zoster = Epstein-Barr virus.

Cytomegalovirus (CMV) is not practically affected.

Uses
- Herpes simplex infections
- Herpes zoster
- Chickenpox.

Side Effects
- Stinging and burning sensation (in topical use)
- Emesis
- Renal toxicity (↓ GFR)
- Tremor, disorientation (reversible neurological manifestation).

Ganciclovir
- Similar to acyclovir
- Higher concentration inside CMV infected cells.

Foscarnet
- Inhibits viral DNA polymerase and reverse transcriptase
- Toxicity is high
- It is used for acyclovir-resistant herpes simplex infection and varicella zoster infections in AIDS patients and in CMV retinitis.

Antiretrovirus
- NRTIs: Zidovudine—Prototype; thymidine analog (azidothymidine, AZT).
    - Mechanism of actions—Zidovudine undergoes intracellular phosphorylation → zidovudine triphosphate →↓ viral reverse transcriptase (RNA-dependent DNA polymerase).
    - Adverse drug reactions—Anemia and neutropenia.

Didanosine: Adverse drug reactions—Pancreatitis and peripheral neuropathy.
Stavudine: Adverse drug reactions—Peripheral neuropathy.
Lamivudine: It also inhibits hepatitis B viral DNA polymerase enzyme. Adverse drug reactions—Well-tolerated drug, but abdominal upset, headache, and anorexia may occur.
- NNRTIs:
  - Directly inhibit HIV reverse transcriptase enzyme
  - Indicated in combination regimen for HIV.
- Protease inhibitors (PIs):

Mechanism of Action

These agents inhibit protease enzyme which is involved in production of structural proteins and enzyme →↓ maturation of new viral particles → immature and noninfectious viruses are formed.

Adverse Drug Reactions
- GI intolerance
- Asthenia
- Headache.

HIV Treatment Guidelines

Treatment should be initiated in:
- Symptomatic HIV disease
- Asymptomatic with CD4 count ≤ 200/mL
- HIV-RNA level: > 20,000 copies/mL.

Therapeutic Regimens
- HAART—Highly active antiretroviral therapy with combination of three or more drugs
- Aim-HIV-RNA copies < 50/mL.

Commonly Prescribed Regimens are
New WHO Treatment Guidelines (2013)
The following all HIV positive patients should receive antiretroviral treatment:
- With CD4 cell count ≤ 500 cell/mm^3
- Child patients under 5 years of age
- Pregnant and breastfeeding females
- With active TB and hepatitis B diseases
- 2-NRTIs + 1-PI
- 2-NRTIs + 1-NNRTIs
- 3-NRTIs.

Integumentary System

Prophylaxis of HIV Infection
- Accidental exposure of health professionals to HIV infection—Zidovudine ± other agents
- Pregnant HIV positive women—Zidovudine to the mother.

DRUGS USED IN THE TREATMENT OF LEPROSY

Classifications
- Sulfone—Dapsone
- Phenazine derivative—Clofazimine
- Antituberculosis drugs—Rifampin
- Other antibiotics
  - Ofloxacin, pefloxacin, sparfloxacin
  - Minocycline
  - Clarithromycin.

Dapsone
- Simplest, cheapest, most active and most commonly used drug for MDT.
- Mechanism of action
  - Para-aminobenzoic acid analog
  - Inhibits folate synthetase
  - Leprostatic
  - Resistance—Primary (in untreated patients); secondary (during therapy).
- Pharmacokinetics
  - Absorption after oral route—Good; wide distribution [Cerebrospinal fluid (CSF)—Poor]; 70% plasma protein binding (PPB); concentrated in lepromatous skin.
  - Acetylation and conjugation (glucuronide and sulfate).
  - Enterohepatic circulation; $t_{½} > 24$ h.
- Adverse drug reactions
  - Hemolytic anemia (high in patients with G6PD deficiency)
  - Gastric intolerance
  - Cutaneous reactions
  - Lepra reaction
  - Hepatitis and agranulocytosis (rare).
- Contraindications—Anemia and G6PD deficiency.

Clofazimine
- Leprostatic and anti-inflammatory
- Mechanism of action—Interferes with template function of DNA

- Dapsone resistant *M. leprae* respond to clofazimine
- Drug for multidrug therapy (MDT)
- Valuable in lepra reaction
- Pharmacokinetics—Orally 40–70%, accumulation in tissues (fat), CSF—Poor; t½—70 days.

Adverse Drug Reactions
- Skin
    - Reddish-black discoloration of skin (major)
    - Discoloration of hair and body secretions
    - Dryness of skin and itching
- GI symptoms
    - Enteritis
    - Nausea, anorexia, and weight loss
- Contraindications—Pregnancy and patients with liver and kidney diseases.

Rifampin
- Bactericidal
- 99.99% killed—3–7 days
- Drug for MDT.
  Contraindications—Hepatic and renal dysfunction.

Multidrug Therapy of Leprosy
- Effective (in dapsone resistance)
- Prevention of resistance (dapsone resistance)
- Quick symptomatic relief
- Reduces total duration of therapy.

WHO-1995, MDT Regimen
- Paucibacillary (tuberculoid/borderline tuberculoid) leprosy—For 6 months
    - Rifampin 600 mg once a month
    - Dapsone 100 mg daily.
- Multibacillary (lepromatous, borderline, borderline lepromatous) leprosy—For 24 months
    - Dapsone 100 mg daily
    - Clofazimine 50 mg daily together with clofazimine 300 mg once a month (29 +1 days)
    - Rifampin 600 mg once a month.

CHAPTER 12

Miscellaneous

EMERGENCY MEDICINES

Atropine Sulfate

Dose
- Bradycardia: 0.5 mg IV every 3–5 min, max 0.04 mg/kg
- Organophosphate and carbamate compounds poisoning: 2 mg every 3 min till adequate atropinization.

Indications
- To restore cardiac rate and arterial pressure during anesthesia when vagal stimulation occurs
- To lessen the degree of A-V heart block
- In organophosphorus poisoning.

Nitroglycerin

Dose
- 0.3–0.4 mg sublingual every 5 min → up to three doses
- For cream—Every 6 h
- For transdermal patch—Apply 12 h a day.

Indications
- Angina pectoris
- Congestive heart failure (CHF) associated with acute myocardial infarction (MI)
- Hypertensive crisis.

Morphine Sulfate

Dose
- Oral: 10–30 mg every 4 h controlled release
- 30 mg every 8–12 h
- SC and IM: 10 mg (5–20 mg)/70 kg 4 hourly

- IV: 2.5–15 mg/70 kg of body weight in 4–5 mL water for injection administered over 4–5 min
- Continuous IV infusion: 0.1–1 mg/mL in 5% dextrose by infusion
- Rectal: 10–30 mg 4 hourly.

Indications
- Moderate-to-severe acute and chronic pain
- Preoperative medication
- As an analgesic during anesthesia
- In acute left ventricular failure and myocardial infarction.

Verapamil
Dose
80–120 mg per oral three times a day.

Indications
- Hypertension
- Angina pectoris
- Supraventricular arrhythmia
- Atrial flutter/fibrillation.

Diltiazem
Dose
- Oral: 30–120 mg, three to four times daily or 60–120 mg
- Twice daily as sustained release capsules
- IV: 0.25 mg/kg.

Indications
- Hypertension
- Angina pectoris
- Supraventricular arrhythmia
- Atrial flutter/fibrillation.

Lignocaine/lidocaine
Dose
- Arrhythmia: IV 0.7–1.4 mg/kg. Not more than 200 mg within 1 h period. IM 4–5 mg/kg
- Local anesthesia: As 2% solution.

Indications
- Local anesthesia
- Ventricular arrhythmia.

Amiodarone
Dose
- Recurrent ventricular arrhythmias: Oral—800–1,600 mg/day for 1–2 weeks.
- Paroxysmal supraventricular tachycardia, symptomatic atrial flutter: Oral—600–800 mg/day for 1 month.
- Ventricular dysrhythmias: 150 mg over the first 10 min followed by 360 mg over the next 6 h.

Indications
- Life-threatening recurrent arrhythmias
- Ventricular fibrillation
- Ventricular tachycardia.

Adrenaline/Epinephrine
Dose
- Cardiac arrest: 1 mg IV of 1:10,000 solution every 3–5 min
- Anaphylaxis: 0.1–1 mg SC or IM of 1:1,000 solution
- Asthma: 0.1–0.3 mg SC or IM of 1:10,000 solution
- Refractory bradycardia and hypotension: 2–10 mcg/min.

Indications
- Bronchial asthma
- Bronchitis
- Emphysema
- Cardiac arrest
- Symptomatic bradycardia
- In local anesthesia
- Exercise-induced bronchospasm
- Aspirin overdose
- Tricyclic antidepressant overdose.

Vasopressin
Dose
5 units IM 3–4 hourly.

Indications
- Diabetes insipidus
- Abdominal distention
- Gastrointestinal bleeding
- Esophageal varices.

Miscellaneous

NaHCO₃
Dose

2-5 mEq/kg IV infusion over 4-8 h.

Indication
- Metabolic acidosis.
- Aspirin overdose
- Tricyclic antidepressant (TCA) overdose

Sodium Nitroprusside
Dose

0.25-0.3 mcg/kg/min.

Indications
- Hypertensive crisis
- To produce controlled hypotension
- To reduce preload and afterload in cardiogenic shock.

Furosemide
Dose
- Pulmonary edema: 40 mg IV
- Edema: 20-80 mg orally everyday in the morning
- Acute congestive heart failure (CHF): Initial dose - 20 to 40 mg IV (slowly over 1 to 2 minutes) or IM once, repeat after 2 hours if required; maintenance dose - 40 mg per oral twice a day.

Indications
- Acute pulmonary edema
- Edema
- Acute CHF.

Mannitol
Dose
- Test dose for marked oliguria or suspected inadequate renal function: 200 mg/kg or 12.5 g as a 15-20% IV solution over 3-5 min, response is adequate if 30-50 mL of urine/h is adequate, a second dose is given if still no response after second dose, stop the drug
- Oliguria: 50 over 90 min to several hours
- Intraocular or intracranial pressure: 1.5-2 g/kg as a 15-20% IV solution over 30-60 min
- Forced diuresis: 10-20% solutions up to 200 g IV.

Indications
- Test dose for marked oliguria or suspected inadequate renal function
- Oliguria
- To induced intraocular or intracranial pressure
- Diuresis in drug intoxication.

Naloxone Hydrochloride
Dose
- Opioid poisoning: 0.4–2 mg IV, IM, and SC repeat doses every 2–3 min as needed
- For postoperative opioid depression: 0.01–0.2 mg IV every 2–3 min, as needed.

Indications
- Opioid poisoning
- For postoperative opioid depression.

Ipecac Syrup
Dose
25–30 mL with water.

Indications
- Poisoning
- Drug overdose.

Activated Charcoal
Dose
30–100 g with water.

Indications
- Poisoning
- Do not mix with ipecac syrup.

Flumazenil
Dose
2 mL IV.

Indication
- Benzodiazepines overdose.

Dopamine

Dose
2–5 mcg/kg/min by IV.

Indications
- In cardiogenic shock (drug of choice, as it also dilates renal vasculature).
- In CHF.

Dobutamine

Dose
0.5–1 mcg/kg/min IV infusion, titrating to optimum dose of 2–20 mcg/kg/min.

Indication
- In acute CHF (drug of choice).

Glucagon

Dose
0.5–1 mg SC, IV, and IM, repeat in 20 minutes as needed.

Indication
- β-blockers overdose.

Salbutamol/Albuterol

Dose
2–4 mg oral; 0.025–0.5 mg IM/SC; 100–200 mcg by inhalation.

Indications
- Asthma
- Prevention of exercise induced spasms.

Diphenhydramine Hydrochloride

Dose
25–50 mg PO, IV, or IM bid/tid.

Indications
- Allergic reactions
- Motion sickness
- Cough suppression
- Sedation.

IMMUNOMODULATORS

Immunomodulator—Substance that helps to regulate the immune system.

Drugs used to modulate the immune response in two ways:
1. Immunosuppression
2. Immunostimulation.

Immunosuppression

- It is used to dampen the immune response in organ transplantation and autoimmune disease.
- Major classes of immunosuppressive drugs used in transplantations
    - Calcineurin inhibitors
    - Antiproliferative and antimetabolite drugs
    - Antibodies
    - Glucocorticoids.

Calcineurin Inhibitors

- The most effective immunosuppressive drugs
- Cyclosporine and tacrolimus
- They target intracellular signaling pathway induced as a consequence of T-cell receptor activation.

Mechanism of Actions

- Cyclosporine/tacrolimus bind to an immunophilin (cyclophilin for cyclosporine/FKBP for tacrolimus), resulting in subsequent interaction with calcineurin to block its phosphatase activity.
- Which is required for the movement of a component of the nuclear factor of activated T-lymphocytes (NFAT) into the nucleus, NFAT in turn is required to induce a number of cytokine genes, including that for IL-2, a prototype T-cell growth, and differentiation factor.

Indication (Cyclosporine)

- Kidney, liver, heart, and other organ transplantation, rheumatoid arthritis, and psoriasis.
- Cyclosporine is usually combined with other agents especially glucocorticoids and either azathioprine or mycophenolate mofetil and most recently sirolimus.
- Rheumatoid arthritis in severe cases that have not responded to methotrexate.
- Psoriasis, Behçet's acute ocular syndrome.

Miscellaneous

Toxicity
- Nephrotoxicity and hepatotoxicity
- Tremor, hirsutism, hypertension, hyperlipidemia, gum hypertrophy and hyperuricemia.

Antiproliferative and Antimetabolite Drugs

Sirolimus/Everolimus

Mechanism of Action
- Sirolimus inhibits T-lymphocytes activation and proliferation.
- It binds to FKBP-12 and the complex inhibits a proteins kinase, mTOR and blocks cell cycle progression at the G1-S phase transition.
- mTOR-mammalian target of rapamycin, a protein kinase that activates Cdks.

Indications
Prophylaxis of organ transplant rejection in combination with a calcineurin inhibitor and glucocorticoid.

Toxicity
- Dose-dependent increase in serum cholesterol and triglyceride.
- Anemia, leukopenia, thrombocytopenia, hypokalemia.
- Fever and gastrointestinal symptoms.

Antimetabolites

Azathioprine
- It is converted to 6-mercaptopurine, which then undergoes further transformation to inhibit de novo purine synthesis.
- It inhibits differentiation and function of T-lymphocytes and inhibits cytolytic lymphocytes.
- Cell-mediated immunity is primarily depressed.

Methotrexate
- Folate antagonist → inhibits cytokine production and cellular immunity.
- Potent immunosuppressant.
- As a first line immunosuppressant in rheumatoid arthritis, pemphigus, myasthenia gravis, etc. Others—Cyclophosphamide and chlorambucil.

Antibodies

Both polyclonal and monoclonal antibodies against lymphocyte cell surface antigen are widely used for prevention and treatment of organ transplant rejection.

Miscellaneous

Polyclonal Antibodies

Generated by repeated injection of human thymocytes [antithymocyte globulin (ATG)] or lymphocyte [antilymphocyte globulin (ALG)] into animals.

Clinical Uses of Monoclonal Antibodies

Monoclonal antibody	Clinical uses and target proteins
Abciximab	Antiplatelet-antagonist of IIb/IIIa (glycoprotein receptors on platelets for fibrinogen); e.g. in unstable angina
Infliximab	Rheumatoid arthritis and Crohn's disease—binds TNFα
Adalimumab	Rheumatoid arthritis—binds to TNFα
Trastuzumab	Breast cancer—binds to HER2 (ERB-B_2)
Daclizumab	Kidney transplants- blocks IL-2 receptors
Muromonab CD3	Kidney transplant—blocks CD3 receptors and prevents allograft rejection
Palivizumab	Respiratory syncytial virus (RSV)—blocks RSV protein
Rituximab	Non-Hodgkin's lymphoma—binds to CD20 of B cells

(HER2 = Human epidermal growth factor receptor 2)

Glucocorticoids

- Prednisolone, methylprednisolone
- Key role in organ transplantation.

Mechanism of Actions

- Suppress cell-mediated immunity and act by inhibiting genes that code for cytokines, IL-1, 2, 3, 4, 5, 6, 8 and TNF-γ, the most important of which is IL-2.
- Inhibit MHC expression.

Immunostimulation

Substances that stimulate the immune system by inducing activation and increasing activity of any of its components.

Two Categories

1. Specific immunostimulator—Antigenic immune specificity, e.g. vaccines.

2. Nonspecific immunostimulator—Acts by irrespective of antigenic specificity
   - Levamisole
     - Originally developed as antihelminthic, restores depressed immune function of B and T-lymphocytes, monocytes and macrophases.
     - Only clinical indication is as adjuvant therapy with 5-FU after surgical resection in patients with colon cancer.
   - Thalidomide
     - It is indicated in treatment of erythema nodosum leprosum and is also used in conditions such as multiple myeloma.
     - Mechanism of action is unclear.
   - Recombinant cytokines—Interferons, INF-α2b, INF-γ-1b, INF-β-1a.

Immunization

Vaccines
Immunoglobulins
[Refer to the chapter on vaccines and antisera].

DRUG-FOOD AND DRUG-DRUG INTERACTIONS

Important Drug-Food Interactions

- Warfarin + high protein diet →↑ albumin→↑ warfarin binding→↓ warfarin effect, i.e. thromboembolic events may occur (e.g. stroke, MI, etc.) (↓ in INR: international normalized ratio).
- Warfarin + vegetables containing vit K/green leafy vegetables/ charcoal broiled meat or food → ↓ warfarin effect, i.e. thromboembolic events may occur (e.g. stroke, MI, etc.) [↓ in INR (international normalized ratio)].
- Warfarin + cooked onions/cranberry juice/grapefruit juice → ↑warfarin effect (↑ INR) → ↑ bleeding.
- Monoamine oxidase inhibitors (moclobemide, selegiline) + tyramine containing food or beverages (cheese, beer, red wine, soy sauce, fermented meats or summer sausages, sauces containing fish or shrimp, aged chicken liver, sauerkraut) → hypertensive crisis (very high BP).
- Theophylline + high-fat meal/grape fruit juice/caffeine (high consumption of coffee) →↑ theophylline toxicity (cardiac arrhythmias).

Miscellaneous

- Antibacterial agents (fluoroquinolones, tetracyclines, etc.) + milk or dairy products → ↓ absorption → ↓ effects (antibiotic failure).

Important Drug Interactions with Ethanol (Alcohol)
- Warfarin + alcohol (acute intoxication) → ↑ warfarin toxicity (bleeding).
- Paracetamol (acetaminophen) + alcohol → ↑ risk of liver damage.
- NSAIDs + alcohol → ↑ risk of GI bleeding/pain and liver damage.
- Diazepam/alprazolam/antihistamines [with central nervous system (CNS) depressants] + alcohol → ↑ CNS depression.
- Insulin + alcohol (acute intoxication) → ↑ risk of hypoglycemia.
- Disulfiram + alcohol → disulfiram reactions (nausea, vomiting, dizziness, throbbing headache, chest tightness and pain, abdominal discomfort, etc.).
- Cephalosporins (cefamandole, cefoperazone, cefotetan, and moxalactam) + alcohol → disulfiram like reactions.
- Metronidazole + alcohol → disulfiram like reactions.
- Sulfonylureas (oral antidiabetic or hypoglycemic agents) + alcohol → ↑ risk of hypoglycemia.
- Chlorpropamide (a sulfonylurea) + alcohol → disulfiram like reactions; ↑ risk of hypoglycemia.

Important Drug-Drug Interactions

Remember
Enzyme inducers (mnemonic: **St. John's wort** **A**nd **B**arbiturates **S**timulate **E**nzyme **R**eaction → **St. John's wort**, **A**nticonvulsants (phenytoin, carbamazepine), **B**arbiturates, **S**moking, **E**thanol, **R**ifampin) increase the metabolism of many drugs and inhibit their effects (assuming that metabolism inactivates a drug and this is not applicable for pro-drugs).

Enzyme inhibitors (mnemonic: **Grapefruit juice** **I**nhibits **COKE V**ery mu**C**h → **Grapefruit juice,** protease inhibitors (**I**ndinavir), **C**imetidine, **O**meprazole, **K**etoconazole, **E**rythromycin, **V**alproic acid/**V**erapamil, **C**iprofloxacin) inhibit the metabolism of many drugs and increase their effects (assuming that metabolism inactivates a drug, and this is not applicable for pro-drugs).

Important examples of drug-drug interactions are as follows:
- Allopurinol + warfarin → ↑warfarin toxicity (bleeding).
- Allopurinol + azathioprine → ↑azathioprine toxicity (bone marrow suppression).

Miscellaneous

- Allopurinol + mercaptopurine → ↑mercaptopurine toxicity.
- Antacids + digoxin/indinavir/iron/itraconazole/ketoconazole/quinolones/aspirin/tetracyclines/L-thyroxine/atazanavir → antacids ↓ effects of the drugs.
- Beta blockers (e.g. propranolol) + selective serotonin reuptake inhibitors (e.g. fluoxetine) → ↑ effects of beta blockers.
- Beta blockers + NSAIDs → ↓ antihypertensive effects of beta blockers.
- Beta blockers + insulin → ↑ risk of hypoglycemia, obliteration of hypoglycemic symptoms (except sweating).
- Beta blockers + sulfonylureas → ↑ risk of hypoglycemia.
- Bile acid sequestrants (bile acid-binding agents) + paracetamol (acetaminophen)/digoxin/furosemide/thiazide diuretics/L-thyroxin → ↓ effects of drugs (due to decreased absorption).
- Erythromycin/clarithromycin + theophylline → ↓ metabolism of theophylline → ↑ risk of theophylline toxicity (cardiac arrhythmias).
- HMG-CoA reductase inhibitors (statins) + clarithromycin/erythromycin/indinavir/rifampin/St. John's wort/verapamil → ↓ metabolism of statins → ↑ risk of myopathy.
- Iron + fluoroquinolones/tetracyclines/L-thyroxine → iron ↓ absorption of the drugs → ↓ effects.
- NSAIDSs + ACE inhibitors/angiotensin receptor blockers/thiazides/furosemide → ↓ antihypertensive and other effects of drugs.
- Oral contraceptive pills (OCPs) containing estrogen + ampicillin/amoxicillin → ↓ enterohepatic circulation of estrogen→ failure of OCPs.
- OCPs containing estrogen + griseofulvin/phenytoin/rifampin/St. John's wort → ↑ metabolism→ failure of OCPs.
- Potassium sparing diuretic agents (spironolactone, amiloride, triamterene) + potassium supplements → hyperkalemia → cardiac arrhythmias.
- Probenecid + methotrexate/penicillins/cephalosporins → decrease renal excretion of the drugs → ↑ effects.
- Probenecid + aspirin → ↓uricosuric effect of probenecid.
- Fluoroquinolones (e.g. ciprofloxacin) + sucralfate → ↓ absorption of quinolones → ↓ effect of quinolones.
- Fluoroquinolones (e.g. ciprofloxacin) + theophylline → ↓ metabolism of theophylline → ↑ risk of theophylline toxicity (cardiac arrhythmias).

Abbreviations

A

ACE	:	angiotensin converting enzyme
ACTH	:	adrenocorticotropic hormone
ADH	:	antidiuretic hormone
AF	:	atrial fibrillation
AFl	:	atrial flutter
AIDS	:	acquired immunodeficiency syndrome
AP	:	action potential
AT1	:	angiotensin receptor 1
ATP	:	adenosine triphosphate
A-V block	:	atrioventricular block
AZT	:	zidovudine (azidothymidine)

B

BAL	:	British antilewisite
BMI	:	body mass index
BP	:	blood pressure
BPH	:	benign prostatic hyperplasia
BZDs	:	benzodiazepines

C

cAMP	:	cyclic adenosine monophosphate
CCBs	:	calcium channel blockers
CD	:	cluster of differentiation
Cdks	:	cyclin dependant proteins
cGMP	:	cyclic guanosine monophosphate
CHF or CCF	:	congestive heart failure or congestive cardiac failure
Cl^-	:	chloride
CMI	:	cell mediated immunity

CMV	:	cytomegalovirus
CNS	:	central nervous system
CPR	:	cardiopulmonary resuscitation
CO	:	cardiac out put
COPD	:	chronic obstructive pulmonary disease
COX	:	cyclooxygenase
CSF	:	cerebrospinal fluid
CTZ	:	chemoreceptor trigger zone
CVS	:	cardiovascular system

D

DA	:	dopamine
DAG	:	diacyl glycerol
DHFRase	:	dihydrofolate reductase
DI	:	diabetes insipidus
DM	:	diabetes mellitus
DNA	:	deoxyribonucleic acid

E

ECG	:	electrocardiogram
EDRF	:	endothelium dependent relaxing factor
ESR	:	erythrocyte sedimentation rate
ECT	:	electroconvulsive therapy

F

F	:	female
5-HT	:	5-hydroxytrypatamine (serotonin)
FKBP	:	FK binding protein
FQs	:	fluoroquinolones
FSH	:	follicular stimulating hormone

G

GABA	:	gamma (γ) aminobutyric acid
GH	:	growth hormone
GFR	:	glomerular filtration rate
GHRH	:	growth hormone releasing hormone
GI	:	gastrointestinal

Abbreviations

GIT	:	gastrointestinal tract
GLUT	:	glucose transporter
Gn	:	gonadotropins
GnRH	:	gonadotropin releasing hormone
GPCR	:	G protein coupled receptor
G6PD	:	glucose 6 phosphate dehydrogenase

H

Hb	:	hemoglobin
HCT	:	hematocrit
HF	:	heart failure
HIV	:	human immunodeficiency virus
HMG-CoA	:	3-hydroxy-3-methyl-glutaryl-coenzyme A
HPA	:	hypothalamus-pituitary-adrenal axis
HR	:	heart rate
HTN	:	hypertension

I

ICP	:	intracranial pressure
ICSH	:	interstitial cell stimulating hormone
ICU	:	intensive care unit
IGF	:	insulin like growth factor
IL	:	interleukin
IP3	:	inositol 1, 4, 5- triphosphate
IU	:	international unit
IUD	:	intrauterine device

J

JAK	:	Janus kinase

K

KI	:	potassium iodide

L

LH	:	luteinizing hormone
LTs	:	leukotrienes
LVF	:	left ventricular failure

M

MAO	:	monoamine oxidase
M	:	male
MI	:	myocardial infarction
MSH	:	melanocyte stimulating hormone
MHC	:	major histocompatibility complex
MU	:	million units

N

NA	:	noradrenaline
NE	:	norepinephrine
NMDA	:	N methyl D aspartate
NNRTIs	:	non-nucleoside reverse transcriptase inhibitors
NO	:	nitric oxide
NRTIs	:	nucleoside reverse transcriptase inhibitors
NS	:	normal saline
NSAIDs	:	non-steroidal anti-inflammatory drugs

O

OHD	:	hydroxy Vit D

P

PAF	:	platelet activating factor
PDE-III	:	Phosphodiesterase III
PG	:	prostaglandin
PIs	:	protease inhibitors
PPB	:	plasma protein binding
PPH	:	postpartum haemorrhage
PSVT	:	paroxysmal supraventricular tachycardia
PTH	:	parathyroid hormone (parathormone)
PU	:	propylthiouracil

R

RBC	:	red blood cell
RL	:	ringer lactate
RNA	:	ribonucleic acid
RTIs	:	respiratory tract infections

S

SABE	: subacute bacterial endocarditis
SSRIs	: selective serotonin reuptake inhibitors
STD	: sexually transmitted disease

T

TB	: tuberculosis
THFA	: tetrahydrofolic acid
TNF α	: tissue necrosis factor α
TRH	: thyrotropin releasing hormone
TSH	: thyroid stimulating hormone
TX	: thromboxane

U

U	: unit
UDP	: uridine diphosphate
UTI	: urinary tract infection

V

VF	: ventricular fibrillation
VT	: ventricular tachycardia

W

WHO	: Word Health Organization
WPW syndrome	: Wolff-Parkinson-White syndrome

Bibliography

- Articles accessed through Pubmed Central
- Bennet PN, Brown MJ. Clinical Pharmacology
- BPKIHS Practical Manual
- Brunton LL, Lazo JS, Parker KL. Goodman and Gilman's: The Pharmacological Basis of Therapeutics
- First AID for the USMLE Step 1
- Kaplan Medical USMLE Step 1 Lecture notes
- Katzung BG. Basic and Clinical Pharmacology
- Rang HP, Dale MM, Ritter JM, Moore PK. Pharmacology
- Sharma HL, Sharma KK. Principles of Pharmacology
- Tripathi KD. Essentials of Medical Pharmacology
- WHO. Guide to Good Prescribing. A Practical Manual

EU GSPR Authorised Reprsentative
Logos Europe, 9 rue Nicolas Poussin
1700, La Rochelle, France
Phone: +33 (0) 6 67 93 73 78
E-mail: contact@logoseurope.eu

www.ingramcontent.com/pod-product-compliance
Ingram Content Group UK Ltd.
Pitfield, Milton Keynes, MK11 3LW, UK
UKHW021831140426
5217IPUK00021B/1393